T0192240

Statistics for Pathologists

Statistics for Pathologists

Danny A. Milner Jr., MD, MSc(Epi)
American Society for Clinical Pathology
Chief Medical Officer
Center for Global Health
Chicago, Illinois

Emily E. K. Meserve, MD, MPH
Fellow, Anatomic and Clinical Pathology
Brigham and Women's Hospital
Boston, Massachusetts

T. Rinda Soong, MD, PhD, MPH
Fellow, Women's and Perinatal Pathology
Department of Pathology
Brigham and Women's Hospital
Boston, Massachusetts

Douglas A. Mata, MD, MPH
Resident, Department of Pathology
Brigham and Women's Hospital
Boston, Massachusetts

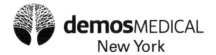
demosMEDICAL
New York

Visit our website at www.demosmedical.com

ISBN: 978-1-6207-0092-1
e-book ISBN: 978-1-6170-5268-2
Data set supplementary materials ISBN: 978-0-8261-8471-9
Data sets provided as an online resource, available at www.demosmedical.com/pathology-data-sets

Acquisitions Editor: David D'Addona
Compositor: diacriTech

Medicine is an ever-changing science. Research and clinical experience are continually expanding our knowledge, in particular our understanding of proper treatment and drug therapy. The authors, editors, and publisher have made every effort to ensure that all information in this book is in accordance with the state of knowledge at the time of production of the book. Nevertheless, the authors, editors, and publisher are not responsible for errors or omissions or for any consequences from application of the information in this book and make no warranty, expressed or implied, with respect to the contents of the publication. Every reader should examine carefully the package inserts accompanying each drug and should carefully check whether the dosage schedules mentioned therein or the contraindications stated by the manufacturer differ from the statements made in this book. Such examination is particularly important with drugs that are either rarely used or have been newly released on the market.

Library of Congress Cataloging-in-Publication Data
Names: Milner, Danny A., Jr. (Danny Arnold), author. | Meserve, Emily E. K.,
    author. | Soong, T. Rinda., author. | Mata, Douglas A., author.
Title: Statistics for pathologists / Danny A. Milner, Jr., MD, American Society for
    Clinical Pathology, Chicago, IL, Emily E.K. Meserve, MD, MPH,
    Brigham and Women's Hospital, Boston, Massachusetts, T. Rinda Soong, MD, PhD,
    MPH, Brigham and Women's Hospital, Boston, Massachusetts, Douglas A. Mata,
    MD, MPH, Brigham and Women's Hospital, Boston, Massachusetts.
Description: New York : Demos Logo, [2017] | Includes bibliographical
    references and index.
Identifiers: LCCN 2016039961 | ISBN 9781620700921 | ISBN 9781617052682 (ebook)
Subjects: LCSH: Diagnosis, Laboratory. | Clinical consultation. |
    Pathologists. | Medicine—Research—Methodology.
Classification: LCC RB37 .M47 2017 | DDC 616.07/56—dc23 LC record available at
    https://lccn.loc.gov/2016039961

Printed in the United States of America by McNaughton & Gunn.

16 17 18 19 20 / 5 4 3 2 1

To Dr. E. Francis (Fran) Cook and Dr. E. John Orav, my first great teachers of statistics
—Danny A. Milner Jr.

To Dr. John Stull
—Emily E. K. Meserve

To Dr. Patti Gravitt and Dr. William Baldwin
—T. Rinda Soong

To my parents, Dr. and Mrs. John and Amy Mata
—Douglas A. Mata

Contents

Preface

Before writing any knowledge-based book, the first question to ask is, "Should this book be written?" Emily, Rinda, and I were motivated to prepare a short course for the United States and Canadian Academy of Pathology (USCAP) annual meeting, by observing the use and misuse of statistical tests in the pathology literature and the frequency with which each of us is approached by colleagues for statistical help. In our opinion, textbooks on statistics and epidemiology are not sufficiently focused, whereas pathology textbooks simply lack information about the application of statistical tests to pathology data sets. In preparing the course syllabus, we reviewed published manuscripts from pathology journals and selected statistical tests and concepts that we saw used regularly in the pathology literature. In defining the scope of our course, we asked ourselves whether pathologists needed to know and understand the concept and execution of statistical testing in order to do their daily jobs. If a pathologist wishes to manage a laboratory, keep up with guideline changes, institute new policies, publish a paper, or convince the finance department to offer a new test, then that pathologist must be able to critically read the literature, documents from product manufacturers, and other sources which contain statistical results (whether used correctly or not). It was within that mind frame that we set out to create a book for pathologists and those working with pathology-based data sets that sits in a middle ground between knowing nothing about statistics and being a savvy statistics guru (i.e., a book for "the rest of us").

Who are we to write such a book? Asking a statistician to write a book for a pathologist would probably have been an okay choice if that statistician spent many years working on pathology studies and data sets, but our fear is the book would still be too heavy on math and theory and too light on practical, hands-on tools. Asking a pathologist to write a book about statistics would probably also be okay, if the author had some working knowledge of the subject. Each coauthor of this book has a degree(s) of some sort that includes statistical training (MPH, PhD, or MSc) and, moreover, uses statistics on a daily basis in research and clinical work. We read pathology journals every month and articles often every day. This provides us with a great deal of insight into what people are doing in the pathology world with statistics (often with the aid of a very advanced nonpathologist statistician), and what tests could and should be understood by all pathologists.

We were greatly aided midway through writing this book by participation in a study with Bob Schmidt, Rachel Factor, and colleagues at the University of Utah/ARUP entitled "Statistical Literacy Among Academic Pathologists," soon to be published in an academic journal, which created, among other great insights, a list of the tests that pathologists should know how to use at a minimum for their practice. We included all of these tests in this book.

What should you know before you read this book? We feel that any pathologist (from first-year residents to senior faculty) should be able to read this book and gain an appreciation if not a set of skills in statistics with no prior knowledge on the subject. Understanding the principles of pathology, as that is used as the thematic focus, is very helpful but not required to find the book useful as the majority of the topics only require understanding of basic science concepts. For the layperson (non-MD), the book is certainly written at a level that could be practically applied to most knowledge bases; however, some of the pathology-focused examples may be confusing. We want it to be clear that this book was written for pathologists by pathologists; however, the kindness and openness of the text should be enjoyable by all.

Data sets to play with are provided in an online resource (available at **www.demosmedical.com/pathology-data-sets**). These data sets are discussed as examples in the text and allow the reader to recreate the statistical processes written about in the text. In most cases, these are real data sets that have been scrubbed, or randomly generated data sets for demonstration purposes. Many of the tests discussed can actually be done in Excel. However, many users will find GraphPad a bit more graphically pleasing. For real power, Stata and/or R remain excellent software for statistics that even a novice can get the hang of quickly with online guides and internal help functions after reading this book.

The one cautionary tale to tell is the same that is told on day 1 of any statistics class. That is, statistics is very much like an old-timey, mad scientist's laboratory with lots of gears, dials, knobs, twisty bits, thingamabobs, and gizmos. A t test may seem simple, but it has assumptions and different formats depending on the input data. In the same way, an elastic net general linear model has presets, assumptions, factors, and settings that can (and should) be adjusted based on exactly what the data are, and how the data set is to be analyzed. This is the fundamental reason we stress over and over again that study design = statistics and statistical analysis = study design. Before picking up the pipette, the syringe, or the scalpel blade, writing out your hypothesis, your plan, and how you will analyze it creates not only a guide and framework, but also checkpoints in your work to keep you honest. The data sets we provide are for your use to practice the application of statistical tests and are a good place to twist the knobs and gizmos to see how they affect the outcome. But, in your own work, these knobs and gizmos have settings that should be dictated from the start of the experiment.

There is a blossoming movement in pathology under the moniker of Molecular Pathoepidemiology (and several variations), which was largely begun by Dr. Shuji Ogino, in Boston. Having worked very closely with Shuji in this field, we also wanted to impart the belief that pathologists who have an understanding of statistics and epidemiological design are better positioned to propose creative hybrid research questions and study designs that intricately amalgamate pathology, epidemiology, and statistical knowledge. These approaches contribute to the development and advancement of personalized medicine. Shuji, my coauthors, and I are strongly encouraging all pathology residency training programs to consider the inclusion of statistical instruction for their trainees, and we feel this book is an excellent starter for that process.

Last, this book is not intended to be a complete guide to statistics, and even the novice reader will see where we have left some gaps that need to be filled through either other courses, books, or consultation with a statistician. There is far too much knowledge in the world we know as well as even more knowledge that we've yet to discover—it's okay to ask for help! But our hope is that by using this book as a tool and guide, you as the pathologist will have the confidence and the courage to conquer the topic.

Danny A. Milner Jr., MD, MSc(Epi)

Acknowledgments

We are indebted to our predecessors and mentors who inspired us and escorted us into the disciplines of statistics and pathology, including Dr. E. Francis Cook, Dr. E. John Orav, Dr. Patti Gravitt, Dr. William Baldwin, and Dr. John Stull to whom this book is being dedicated. We especially appreciate the generous contributions of our colleagues to this book, including Dr. A. Agoston, whose study on esophageal adenocarcinoma supplied the data for our discussion on survival analyses (Chapter 7), and Dr. Scott Tomlins, whose course materials for the American Society for Investigative Pathology (ASIP) 2016 Annual Meeting provided invaluable biologic conceptual frameworks for our case examples in the chapters on comparative statistics and concordance statistics (Chapters 3 and 4).

Last but not least, many thanks to David D'Addona, Norman Graubart, Joseph Stubenrauch, Nandhakumar Krishnan, and the rest of the publishing team whose efforts have been vital to the success of this book.

CHAPTER 1

Introduction to Statistics for Pathologists

Emily E. K. Meserve
Danny A. Milner Jr.

▓ INTRODUCTION

"Statistics" is a term used frequently in many fields with different connotations and different degrees of importance. Listening to a sportscast of baseball in America, the rabid fan is inundated with records (0.356 batting average), numbers (400th strikeout of career), or firsts (first triple play in a World Series since 1972)—each a carefully documented data point being reported as a descriptive statistic. Descriptive statistics similarly captivate the attention of political analysts and citizens in the form of polling data—especially in the 2 years before a presidential election. In political polling discourse, we frequently encounter statements such as "Candidate A is leading polls this week with 23%, followed closely by Candidate B with 21%." The metrics for each example require obsessive and rigorously detailed data collection, but the mathematics used to calculate the statistics and the manner in which these statistics are presented is intuitive. There are many other examples of statistics in everyday life that are used for (among other things): (a) convenience (to summarize an event or topic), (b) desired outcome (to increase the interest of the audience), and/or (c) understanding (to present useful information of value). In the field of medicine, the careful researcher should report statistics primarily for understanding and avoid, at all cost, convenience and desired outcome—"just the facts, please!"

Within medicine, there are different types of statistics used on a daily basis to care for patients, understand human physiology/

pathophysiology, and perform experiments in laboratory settings far removed from the human subject. When medical teams go on rounds and present a differential diagnosis, this is based on statistics (epidemiology of human disease) and refined by the clinical presentation, history, and laboratory data, although rarely would a doctor say, "There is a 34% chance that this patient is having myocardial infarction, followed by a 30% chance of an anxiety attack." However, medical teams must realize that statistical probabilities underlie the composition and ordering of this list. Before administering a treatment regimen, rigorously generated data and statistics have been employed (think FDA-level) to determine that, for example, "Drug A is the best choice for Condition X because in a study of 4,000 people with Condition X, 95% of 2,000 people given Drug A had Benefit 1 without Side Effect α while 85% of 2,000 people given Drug B had Benefit 1 without Side Effect α." Related to this clinical trial, as described, would be a P value for the difference (95% vs. 85%) and an effect size (10% difference). These data may not be verbally discussed in great detail every time the drug is given; however, they will form the basis of why drug A is given instead of drug B, at least until drug C is developed, tested against drug A, and determined to be more beneficial. However, unlike the example of a differential diagnosis (which may represent hundreds if not thousands of studies), clinical trials for drug A versus drug B may only number in the dozens. Another area of medicine that very frequently uses statistics is basic and translational research, where scientists may be dealing with mice, cells in a dish, blood samples from patients, or any number of other in vitro experiments where conditions can be carefully controlled but numbers of subjects are often much smaller. In this setting, the types of data and the exact nature of the comparisons to be performed require careful use of precise statistics to generate hypotheses, test hypotheses, and extrapolate potential benefits to the human population.

One of the most important concepts in statistics and one that most fail to understand early in their academic adventures: study design requires statistics and statistics inform study design. Before the first mouse is injected and before the first cells are plated, the exact statistical tests that are to be used for analysis should be spelled out. Many basic and translational researchers have unfortunately likely found themselves in the situation of having collected data but struggling to know whether and how to perform analysis. These situations highlight the fact that knowledge of basic research design and statistical fundamentals is quintessential to execute valid research investigations in any medical specialty. Primarily, this knowledge gives researchers the freedom to perform accurate initial analyses by selecting appropriate descriptive statistics to report and comparative statistics to perform. Furthermore, a basic knowledge allows researchers to triage situations in which expert statistical skills are necessary and provides a framework and vocabulary for discussions with these experts.

Pathology, as the founding principle or definition of a given disease, is a medical specialty, which naturally flows from the basic science lab through translational research and into clinical medicine. As such, understanding knowledge acquired at all three levels and being confident in the importance and significance of such findings in the reality of patients (as opposed to the restricted universe of an experiment) is paramount to making lifesaving discoveries while doing no harm. Sadly, research design and statistical fundamentals are a relatively minor component of most medical school curricula and are often nearly absent from pathology residency training. This lack of knowledge coupled with the nature of common study designs in pathology is a significant challenge for conducting valid statistical analyses. Often in surgical pathology, studies are small convenience samples usually due to investigation of a rare diagnosis, or the type of data may be difficult to determine, such as count versus continuous data, or the distribution of the variable in the population may not be known, thus requiring consideration of alternative, less familiar statistical methods.

As surgical pathologists with statistical training, we regularly receive questions from colleagues about how best to perform statistical analysis of data. We are also aware of common situations in pathology research that are problematic and often lead to erroneous use of statistical methods. In this book, we cover basic statistical fundamentals and selected additional topics within the context of pathology-specific application. We hope that this approach will serve as a guide to understanding and performing basic descriptive tests, avoiding common pitfalls, and initiating additional conversations about more complicated analyses with local statistical experts.

Chapter 2 starts with discussion of exploratory data analyses and descriptive statistics. This includes preanalytic visual examination of data sets and individual variables using tabulation and graphing as well as data checking to identify missing or erroneous values. These steps apply to any kind of data and are necessary in any study design before further analysis to ensure the data set is complete and robust. Additionally, exploratory data analyses and descriptive statistics help guide selection of appropriate statistical tests for use in subsequent analysis. This chapter concludes with methods by which relationships between two variables can be described, again to better understand the distributions of variables within the data set and to identify related variables, thus helping to guide subsequent statistical analysis.

Ex. What is the average (mean) gestational age at delivery in a random sample of 118 histologically unremarkable placentas?

The data can be visually examined with a histogram (see Figure 1.1, using Excel), and descriptive statistics such as mean (38 weeks, 4 days), median (39 weeks, 1 day), mode (37 weeks, 0 days), standard deviation (2.05), skewness (−0.96), and kurtosis (0.93) can be calculated. Initial visual examination of the histogram and descriptive statistics suggest that the data have a negative skew but that it is reasonable to use comparative statistics in subsequent analysis that assume an underlying normal distribution for this variable.

Chapter 3 includes discussion of the most fundamental comparative statistics that are widely used in data analysis. This chapter begins with basic definitions of important concepts in performing and interpreting statistical tests and continues with discussion of parametric and nonparametric methods, the latter being frequently relevant in pathology studies due to lack of information about the distribution of uncommon or novel variables in the population. Some of the most commonly used statistical tests in pathology studies, including *t* test, analysis of variance (ANOVA), Wilcoxon–Mann–Whitney test, and chi-square and Fisher's exact tests, are discussed in this chapter.

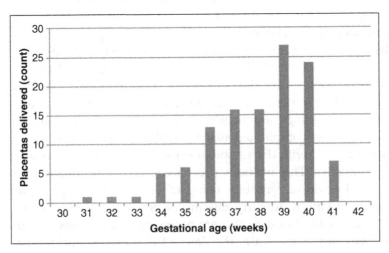

FIGURE 1.1
Histogram describing the distribution of gestational age at delivery in a random sample of 118 histologically normal placentas.

Ex. Is age of presentation with high-grade serous carcinoma (HGSC) different in *BRCA1* germ line mutated women (age_group = 1) compared to *BRCA1* germ line wild-type (age_group = 0)?

Initial descriptive statistics indicate that nonparametric methods should be utilized. Using the Wilcoxon rank-sum test (also known as the Wilcoxon–Mann–Whitney test or the Mann–Whitney U test) in Stata (Figure 1.2), it can be determined that the age of presentation with HGSC is significantly lower in BRCA1 mutated women than age of presentation with HGSC in BRCA1 wild-type women.

Chapter 4 focuses on two types of analysis commonly used in pathology studies: concordance and reproducibility analyses. Concordance analyses are commonly used to evaluate the relatedness between variables, but an important limitation is that these analyses do not yield information about causality or enable prediction. Therefore, careful attention must be given to how the results of concordance analyses are reported so as to not overstate the findings. Several measures used in diagnostic reproducibility studies are then discussed, including percent agreement, intraclass correlation coefficient, and several types of kappa statistics. It is necessary to remember that there are several study design elements (e.g., number of reviewers) that may affect diagnostic reproducibility and subsequently how data sets can be analyzed.

Ex. Two pathologists each review 48 diagnostic cervical biopsies and diagnose either low-grade squamous intraepithelial lesion

```
Two-sample Wilcoxon rank-sum (Mann-whitney) test

   age_group |      obs      rank sum      expected
-------------+------------------------------------------
           0 |       30        995.5          840
           1 |       25        544.5          700
-------------+------------------------------------------
    combined |       55         1540         1540

unadjusted variance          3500.00
adjustment for ties            -7.70
                           ----------
adjusted variance            3492.30

Ho: age(age_gr~p==0) = age(age_gr~p==1)
             z =      2.631
    Prob > |z| =     0.0085
```

FIGURE 1.2
Example Stata output for Wilcoxon rank-sum (Mann–Whitney) test.

(LSIL = outcome 0) or high-grade squamous intraepithelial lesion (HSIL = outcome 1). What is the diagnostic agreement between these two pathologists?

Initial descriptive statistics performed in Stata indicate that, when categorized by the initial diagnosis documented in the surgical pathology report, 79.17% of cases were classified as LSIL and 20.83% of cases were classified as HSIL. However, when comparing agreement between the two reviewers, overall percent agreement was 77.08%. The calculated kappa statistic was 0.2626, indicating only fair agreement between reviewers (Figure 1.3).

Chapter 5 continues with an introduction to regression analysis, including model selection, and then focuses on more detailed discussion of logistic regression, including ordinal logistic regression, and linear regression. Each of these methods can be useful in pathology studies. Notably, ordinal logistic regression could be applied commonly to data sets encountered in pathology because it can be used to analyze variables when the outcome of interest is a categorical variable with more than two categories that have ordered meaning, such as tumor confined to an organ, tumor with spread into adjacent organs, and tumor with distant metastases or reactive atypia, high-grade dysplasia, and invasive adenocarcinoma. In addition to model building, this chapter also details steps for checking the assumptions and fit of the model.

Ex. A data set contains 200 osteosarcomas that have been characterized by the presence or absence of a novel cytogenetic abnormality. Outcome data includes presence or absence of metastasis at 6 months. Other variables include age, gender, history of trauma to affected site, history of cigarette smoking, mitotic count, presence/absence of

outcome	Freq.	Percent	Cum.
0	38	79.17	79.17
1	10	20.83	100.00
Total	48	100.00	

Agreement	Expected Agreement	Kappa	Std. Err.	Z	Prob>Z
77.08%	68.92%	0.2626	0.0723	3.63	0.0001

FIGURE 1.3
Example Stata output for data tabulation and agreement statistics.

necrosis, and size of tumor at presentation. What is the effect of the presence of the cytogenetic abnormality on metastasis? Logistic regression uses a "yes/no" outcome (yes = metastasis vs. no = no metastasis) as the outcome of interests and asks what the effect of the presence (yes) or absence (no) of the cytogenetic abnormality would be. In a simple world, we would just do a Fisher's exact test from the two-by-two table, but the other variables (age, gender, etc.) may also have an effect on rate of metastasis. To determine the true association of the cytogenetic abnormality with metastasis, we need to control for the other variables by including them in a model of logistic regression. Similarly, we may want to predict metastasis from known risk factors, and a logistic regression model can work in the same way.

In the univariate two-by-two table, we see a strong association (P value ~ .000) and the odds ratio would be 9.0 (very strong effect) (Figure 1.4A). What happens when we control for all variables? We see a similar odds ratio for the cytogenetic abnormality (11.3) and values for the other variables, which are not significant (not P values for each variable in the model). With model selection, we can reduce the important effects to just cytogenetics and mitotic rate (Figure 1.4B). Note, throughout, the odds ratio for cytogenetic abnormality does not drastically change, which CAN occur during model selection (indicating the importance of strong covariates).

met	cyto 0	1	Total
0	76	25	101
1	25	74	99
Total	101	99	200

```
            Pearson chi2(1) =   49.9900   Pr = 0.000
    likelihood-ratio chi2(1) =   52.3115   Pr = 0.000
              Cramér's V =    0.4999
                   gamma =    0.8000   ASE = 0.059
          Kendall's tau-b =    0.4999   ASE = 0.061
          Fisher's exact =             0.000
      1-sided Fisher's exact =             0.000
```

FIGURE 1.4A
Example Stata output for Pearson chi-square and Fisher's exact test.

```
. logistic met cyto age gender traum smoke mit nec size

Logistic regression                              Number of obs   =       200
                                                 LR chi2(8)      =    140.70
                                                 Prob > chi2     =    0.0000
Log likelihood = -68.269356                      Pseudo R2       =    0.5075
```

met	Odds Ratio	Std. Err.	z	P>|z|	[95% Conf. Interval]	
cyto	11.34582	5.31976	5.18	0.000	4.526154	28.44082
age	1.010217	.025031	0.41	0.682	.9623294	1.060488
gender	1.675327	.752076	1.15	0.250	.6949994	4.038453
traum	1.719629	.7758331	1.20	0.230	.7102385	4.163566
smoke	1.442894	.6359775	0.83	0.405	.6082115	3.42306
mit	1.598009	.121547	6.16	0.000	1.376688	1.85491
nec	.6042055	.267831	-1.14	0.256	.2534345	1.440468
size	.9145723	.0732225	-1.12	0.265	.7817523	1.069958

```
. logistic met cyto mit

Logistic regression                              Number of obs   =       200
                                                 LR chi2(2)      =    135.30
                                                 Prob > chi2     =    0.0000
Log likelihood = -70.971671                      Pseudo R2       =    0.4880
```

met	Odds Ratio	Std. Err.	z	P>|z|	[95% Conf. Interval]	
cyto	10.25884	4.573163	5.22	0.000	4.282048	24.57791
mit	1.556573	.1101253	6.25	0.000	1.355028	1.788096

FIGURE 1.4B
Example Stata output for logistic regression model.

Chapter 6 starts with a discussion of count data, a seemingly intuitive though often misunderstood concept in statistics and in pathology. Count data are most easily thought of as variables for which the increment of measure cannot be meaningfully subdivided. A practical pathology example includes mitotic count—pathologists count 5 or 6 mitoses but this increment of measure is not meaningfully subdivided into 5.25 or 5.6 mitoses. The important aspect of count data is that it always has a denominator (mitoses per 10 hpf). Therefore, although one may count in only whole numbers, the *rate* may be a fractional quantity (5.6 mitosis per 10 hpf). Specifically, Poisson statistics evaluate count data, so the chapter continues with discussion and practical examples of the use of the Poisson distribution and statistics for analysis of count data relevant to pathologists. Comparison with other similar methods and when to use which are provided.

Ex. A large data set of patients with acral lentiginous melanoma presenting from in situ to invasive ($n = 45$) is collected, which includes the number of metastases observed in any site during the first year after diagnosis (count over time) as well as depth of invasion, age, gender, and margins status. A subset of the patients received chemotherapy. What was the effect of having chemotherapy (vs. not) on the evolution of metastases?

Similar to the earlier logistic regression, Poisson regression for the dependent variable of number of metastases over 1 year shows a strong negative correlation with the presence of chemotherapy (counts were smaller in patients who received chemotherapy) when controlled for other variables (Figure 1.5). Note that in this version of the model, positive margins are also negatively correlated and significant. However, after model variable selection, only chemotherapy remains as significant.

Chapter 7 focuses on survival analyses and begins with an introduction to time-to-event data using pathology-focused examples. This introduction also includes discussion of the concept of censoring as related to study designs commonly encountered in pathology research. The chapter follows with a discussion of Kaplan–Meier analyses along with detailed examples. Finally, the chapter discusses the available models for survival analyses with special focus on using Cox proportional hazards model.

Ex. A sample of 52 women with high-grade serous carcinoma (HGSC) of the ovary/fallopian tube is assembled. Mutation status of *BRCA1* and *BRCA2* is determined. Additionally, data are collected on whether the patient is alive or dead of disease at last known follow-up and length of time to last known follow-up (months). Performing a Kaplan–Meier survival analysis can determine whether *BRCA1/2*

```
Poisson regression                          Number of obs   =        45
                                            LR chi2(5)      =     66.58
                                            Prob > chi2     =    0.0000
Log likelihood = -124.0186                  Pseudo R2       =    0.2116
```

nummets	Coef.	Std. Err.	z	P>|z|	[95% Conf. Interval]	
chemo	-1.114371	.1584907	-7.03	0.000	-1.425007	-.8037348
depthmm	.0368636	.0304232	1.21	0.226	-.0227649	.096492
age	.0000328	.004322	0.01	0.994	-.0084381	.0085038
gender	.0692164	.1088614	0.64	0.525	-.144148	.2825808
posmargs	-.2340524	.1112059	-2.10	0.035	-.452012	-.0160927
_cons	2.3773	.2093336	11.36	0.000	1.967014	2.787587

FIGURE 1.5
Example Stata output for Poisson regression.

mutation status confers survival advantage or disadvantage in this sample (Figure 1.6).

Chapter 8 introduces and discusses classification and clustering analysis. These techniques are used commonly, for example, in studies to show relationships between strains of bacteria or when attempting to identify diagnostic immunohistochemistry algorithms. The chapter highlights several different techniques, including classification and regression tree analysis (CART®, Salford Systems). It continues with an introduction to clustering analyses that includes supervised and unsupervised techniques as well as differential expression analysis.

Ex. A new laboratory planned to implement immunohistochemistry. Working within certain cost constraints, the laboratory decided to undertake a study to determine which immunohistochemical markers can be used in algorithmic fashion to optimize diagnosis of hematolymphoid malignancies that appear on routine hematoxylin and eosin (H&E) stain as medium-sized/large cells in tissue sections. All available immunohistochemical data were collected from surgical pathology

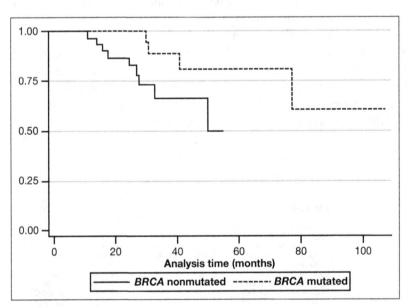

FIGURE 1.6
Example Stata output of a Kaplan–Meier curve. In analysis of this small sample, there was no significant difference in survival for women with *BRCA1/2* mutation compared to those without *BRCA1/2* mutation (*P* > .05).

reports on 91 leucocyte common antigen (LCA)-positive cases with the morphologic features of interest. Missing data were imputed as needed by expert opinion (see Chapter 9).

Using CART, multiple decision trees were generated using various combinations of immunohistochemical stained slides. A representative branch of one decision tree is shown in Figure 1.7. Sensitivity analyses were performed. Ultimately, the decision tree with the fewest number of decision points

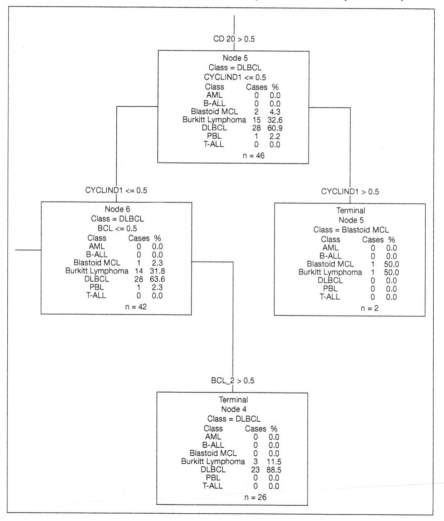

FIGURE 1.7

Example of classification and regression tree analysis output (redrawn based on original CART, Salford Systems output).

(i.e., immunostains to include in the algorithm panel) that generated the fewest ambiguous classifications (i.e., relative error) was selected. The final algorithm additionally required a single additional confirmatory immunostain.

Chapter 9 covers concepts and strategies related to sample size and "missing data." Missing data occur when it is not practical or possible to collect a value for every variable for each individual in the data set. In pathology, when conducting prospective studies this may be due to prohibitive cost or other resource limitation. However, more often, pathologists encounter missing data when performing retrospective studies wherein perhaps a particular immunostain of interest was performed on some but not all cases or when patients are lost to follow-up and clinical outcome cannot be completely documented for all patients. Therefore, Chapter 9 focuses discussion on how to determine the effect that missing data have on a data set, whether and how the data set can be salvaged, including methods for imputation, as well as suggestions for when to consider simply gathering more data (i.e., recruiting more individuals to the data set or acquiring resources to perform the missing immunostains).

Ex. A data set is given to you that contains 1,000 patients with rheumatoid nodules (current or in the past) who also have a malignancy (*n* = 400) along with patients with rheumatoid nodules with no history of malignancy (*n* = 600) (Figure 1.8). In addition to age, gender,

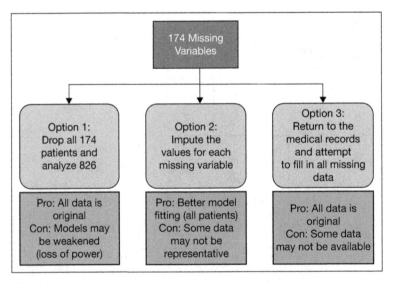

FIGURE 1.8
Flowchart describing options for handling missing data.

drug regimen, type of cancer, stage, smoking history, and a battery of 20+ laboratory results, expression data (RNAseq) from rheumatoid nodules and the tumors are available with confirmatory RT-PCR on a set of 13 candidate genes. In perusing the data, you note that age is missing for 18 patients, gender is missing for 2 patients, drug regimen is missing for 10 patients, smoking history is missing for 24 patients, and at least one of the 20 lab tests is missing for 120 patients. There is, sadly, no overlap in the missing data (each patient is missing only one piece of data). In total, 174 patients have incomplete data for variables other than cancer and expression. The missing data are evenly split between cases and controls. How would you approach this missing data? (See Figure 1.8.)

■ COMMENTS REGARDING STATISTICAL SOFTWARE

There are multiple software packages that can be used for data analysis. Microsoft Excel has basic statistical functionality and can be useful for initial descriptive and comparative analyses. Several dedicated statistical software packages, including SAS, SPSS, Stata, GraphPad Prism, and CART require individual or institutional purchase. Other packages, such as R, PSPP, or Weka, are available freely online. As a general rule, the freely available statistical packages usually require knowledge of the programming language (or "code") used by the software in order to conduct analysis. On the other hand, packages available for purchase usually have a more user-friendly interface that does not require exact knowledge of the programming language and allows analysis via use of intuitive drop-down menus. SAS is a notable exception wherein users must be familiar with the SAS programming language as well as the fundamental mathematics on which the code is based. Statistical packages, whether available online or for purchase, also now often have websites, documents and/or books, and listservs devoted to assisting and helping users.

■ RECOMMENDED READING

CART
   https://www.salford-systems.com/products/cart
Cuff J, Higgins JP. Statistical analysis of surgical pathology data
   using the R program. *Adv Anat Pathol*. May 2012;19(3):131-139.
   doi:10.1097/PAP.0b013e318254d842

GraphPad

 http://www.graphpad.com

R

 https://www.r-project.org

SAS

 http://www.sas.com/en_us/learn/analytics-u.html#software

SPSS

 http://www-01.ibm.com/software/analytics/spss/products/
 statistics

Stata

 http://www.stata.com/support/faqs

 http://www.statalist.org

 href="http://www.ats.ucla.edu/stat/stata

Weka

 http://www.cs.waikato.ac.nz/ml/weka

CHAPTER 2

Exploratory Data Analysis and Descriptive Statistics

Douglas A. Mata
Danny A. Milner Jr.

■ INTRODUCTION

Like most pathologists, we often find ourselves in the following situation. We have a spreadsheet full of data—be it from a retrospective chart review, a prospective cohort study, or a randomized clinical trial—and a list of questions that we want to ask of it. If we are a typical physician, we are likely excited at the prospect of getting down to business and performing statistical analyses to test our hypotheses. Before doing so, a warning: do not get ahead of ourselves, or we risk committing a major error. Before even thinking about making inferences from our data using a litany of t tests, chi-square tests, and regression models, the best approach is to take a moment to look at and better appreciate our data. This chapter offers instruction in descriptive statistics. Before making inferences using a data set, let's first look at and describe our variables.

■ OUR EXAMPLE

In order to get the best use of this chapter, it is useful to start directly with the descriptive analysis of an example data set. We have collected information on 100 individuals who were diagnosed with kidney cancer. We have painstakingly typed this information into a spreadsheet in which every row represents a single patient and every column represents a variable. For this chapter, we will use a spreadsheet with basic demographic, operative, and pathologic data on 100 patients who underwent nephrectomy for a renal mass. These data are available to us in the file entitled "chapter2.csv" (**online materials; available at www.demosmedical.com/pathology-data-sets**) and can be opened in Microsoft Excel or the spreadsheet program of your choosing. Please note that there are two sheets in this file. The first is our data (Raw Data) and the second is the data dictionary (Data Dictionary). Let's start with the data dictionary, which is an excellent tool to always include in a data set, especially when it is to be shared or public. There are seven variables in the data set for each patient, the first of which is our unique identifier. In addition, we have the patient's gender and age as well as details of the surgery and the tumor itself. Now that we have a grasp of what our variables are, let's look at each in raw detail.

What kind of variables might we have? In our data set, the first three columns contain demographic information: a patient identifier, the gender of the patient, and the age at surgery (Figure 2.1). The fourth and fifth columns contain operative information: the side of the surgery and the type of surgery. Last, the sixth and seventh columns contain pathologic information: the size and stage of the tumor. In a more complete data set, we might also have information on other variables such as patient body mass index, the name of the surgeon performing the operation, the grade of the tumor, and treatment outcomes. This simpler spreadsheet will serve for illustrative purposes for now. Note that the basic description of our data was in the data dictionary, but when we look at the data we can get a sense of the variability by eye instantaneously.

Loading the Data Into R

Before we look at our data by creating some simple graphs and computing some basic descriptive statistics, we need to load it into the software program that we will use to perform our analyses. In this chapter, we have three programs. The first is the free statistical analysis program known as R, which is available for both Windows and Macintosh (R Project for Statistical Computing, Vienna, Austria).[1] Once R is installed, double-click on the R icon to open up the console, shown in Figure 2.2.

---

[1] Available for download at www.r-project.org

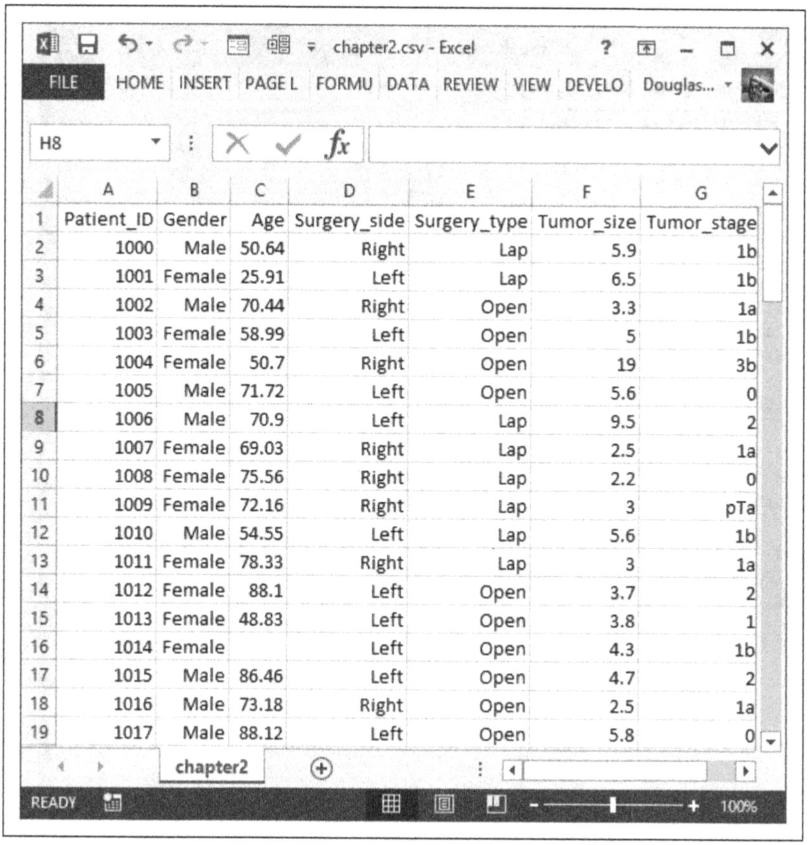

Patient_ID	Gender	Age	Surgery_side	Surgery_type	Tumor_size	Tumor_stage
1000	Male	50.64	Right	Lap	5.9	1b
1001	Female	25.91	Left	Lap	6.5	1b
1002	Male	70.44	Right	Open	3.3	1a
1003	Female	58.99	Left	Open	5	1b
1004	Female	50.7	Right	Open	19	3b
1005	Male	71.72	Left	Open	5.6	0
1006	Male	70.9	Left	Lap	9.5	2
1007	Female	69.03	Right	Lap	2.5	1a
1008	Female	75.56	Right	Lap	2.2	0
1009	Female	72.16	Right	Lap	3	pTa
1010	Male	54.55	Left	Lap	5.6	1b
1011	Female	78.33	Right	Lap	3	1a
1012	Female	88.1	Left	Open	3.7	2
1013	Female	48.83	Left	Open	3.8	1
1014	Female		Left	Open	4.3	1b
1015	Male	86.46	Left	Open	4.7	2
1016	Male	73.18	Right	Open	2.5	1a
1017	Male	88.12	Left	Open	5.8	0

FIGURE 2.1
The first few rows of our data set shown in Microsoft Excel. We can scan down each column and see, to some degree, the inherent variability in the data, but formal tests are still needed.

Now that we have installed and opened R, we can load our example data by typing the following code into the command prompt. This code saves our spreadsheet as an "object" in R's memory known as a "data frame." We will name our data frame df. This is the name that we will type into the command prompt in order to access our spreadsheet from within R.

```
# Import chapter two example data into R
df <- read.csv("chapter2.csv", header = TRUE)
```

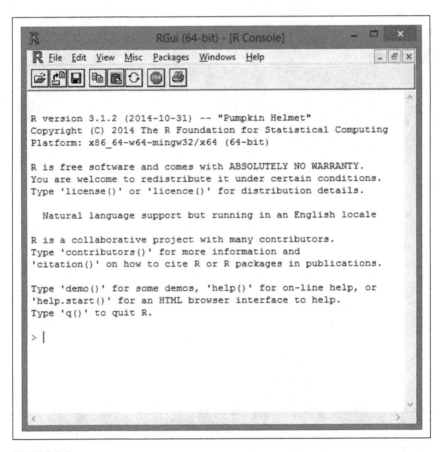

FIGURE 2.2
The R console has standard drop-down menus, quick reference buttons, and then the command line where all programming language can be entered for analysis.

Loading the Data Into Stata

As long as our data is in a spreadsheet where the variables are across the tops of the columns and each row represents a study subject, importing the data requires only that we copy and paste it into the data editor. The icon for the data editor is a button at the top of the screen (Figure 2.3) and requires only that we confirm that the top row either is or is not variable names. Our data is now ready for analysis.

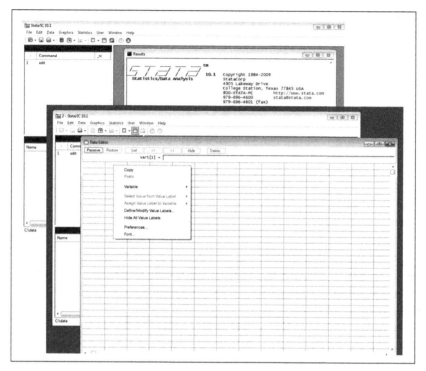

FIGURE 2.3
The Stata console, which, like R, has drop-down menus, quick reference buttons, and a command line for entering code.

■ GETTING ORIENTED

You saw what our spreadsheet looked like in Microsoft Excel in Figure 2.1. From Excel, we know that we have 100 rows of patient records along with seven variables. This entire spreadsheet is represented within R as df. We can confirm that df matches the dimensions of our Excel file by typing the following code:

```
# Check dimensions of the data frame
> dim(df)
[1] 100 7
```

After confirming that, we can visually inspect the first few rows of our spreadsheet by using the head() command. If you want to instead look at the bottom few rows, you could instead use the tail() command. Give both a try.

```
# Peek at first six rows of our data frame
> head(df)
Patient_ID Gender Age Surgery_side Surgery_type Tumor_
size Tumor_stage
1  1000  Male    50.64  Right  Lap    5.9   1b
2  1001  Female  25.91  Left   Lap    6.5   1b
3  1002  Male    70.44  Right  Open   3.3   1a
4  1003  Female  58.99  Left   Open   5.0   1b
5  1004  Female  50.70  Right  Open  19.0   3b
6  1005  Male    71.72  Left   Open   5.6    0
```

There you have it. Our data frame, df, is now loaded into R. Every row is a patient. Every column is a variable. If we had our data set open in Excel and wanted to select a particular variable, we could simply highlight the column of interest as in Figure 2.4.

We can do the same thing in R by attaching the dollar sign operator to the name of our data frame df. This technique is a powerful tool as it allows us to manipulate our variables in vector form.

```
# Print a vector of the ID numbers of all patients
> df$Patient_ID
1000 1001 1002 1003 1004 1005 1006 1007 1008 1009 1010
1011 1012 1013 1014 1015 1016 1017 1018 1019 1020 1021
1022 1023 1024 1025 1026 1027 1028 1029 1030 1031 1032
1033 1034 1035 1036 1037 1038 1039 1040 1041 1042 1043
1044 1045 1046 1047 1048 1049 1050 1051 1052 1053 1054
1055 1056 1057 1058 1059 1060 1061 1062 1063 1064 1065
1066 1067 1068 1069 1070 1071 1072 1073 1074 1075 1076
1077 1078 1079 1080 1081 1082 1083 1084 1085 1086 1087
1088 1089 1090 1091 1092 1093 1094 1095 1096 1097 1098
1099
```

In Stata, the command "list" followed by a variable will display all values for a given variable for all patients in a continuous list. Because each patient in our data set contributes one observation, we should have 100 unique patient identifiers. An initial step of any analysis is to check your data set to ensure that it has what you think it has in it. Rather

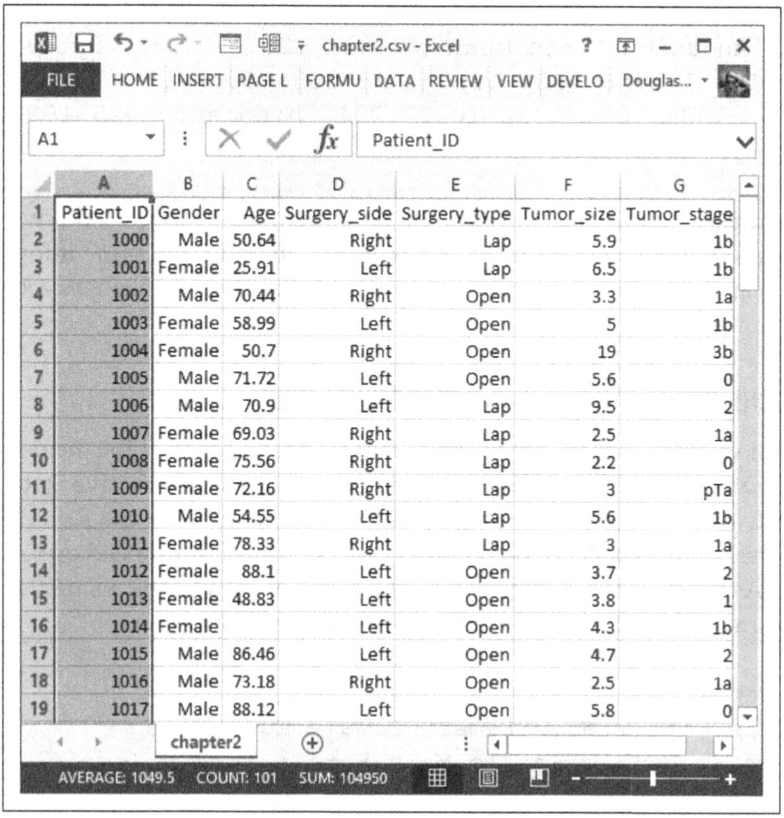

	A	B	C	D	E	F	G
1	Patient_ID	Gender	Age	Surgery_side	Surgery_type	Tumor_size	Tumor_stage
2	1000	Male	50.64	Right	Lap	5.9	1b
3	1001	Female	25.91	Left	Lap	6.5	1b
4	1002	Male	70.44	Right	Open	3.3	1a
5	1003	Female	58.99	Left	Open	5	1b
6	1004	Female	50.7	Right	Open	19	3b
7	1005	Male	71.72	Left	Open	5.6	0
8	1006	Male	70.9	Left	Lap	9.5	2
9	1007	Female	69.03	Right	Lap	2.5	1a
10	1008	Female	75.56	Right	Lap	2.2	0
11	1009	Female	72.16	Right	Lap	3	pTa
12	1010	Male	54.55	Left	Lap	5.6	1b
13	1011	Female	78.33	Right	Lap	3	1a
14	1012	Female	88.1	Left	Open	3.7	2
15	1013	Female	48.83	Left	Open	3.8	1
16	1014	Female		Left	Open	4.3	1b
17	1015	Male	86.46	Left	Open	4.7	2
18	1016	Male	73.18	Right	Open	2.5	1a
19	1017	Male	88.12	Left	Open	5.8	0

FIGURE 2.4
Selecting the patient ID variable in Excel.

than painstakingly reading through the aforementioned printed list to confirm that we have 100 unique patients, you can ask R to double-check it for you. The describe() function from the Hmisc package can be used for this purpose. To install the package, type the following code into the command prompt. You only need to install it once. Next time, when you restart R, simply type library(Hmisc) to load the package.

```
# Install and load the Hmisc package
install.packages("Hmisc")
library(Hmisc)

# Check for number of unique values
> describe(df$Patient_ID)
```

```
df$Patient_ID
n missing unique Info Mean .05 .10 .25 .50 .75 .90 .95
100 0 100 1 1050 1005 1010 1025 1050 1074 1089 1094
lowest: 1000 1001 1002 1003 1004, highest: 1095 1096
1097 1098 1099
```

As previously mentioned, the variable df$Patient_ID does indeed have 100 unique patient identifiers, as we expected. In Stata, the same information can be found for any variable using the "summarize *variable, detail*" command.

■ DESCRIBING AND GRAPHING CATEGORICAL VARIABLES

Now that we have confirmed this basic fact, let's take a look at the gender breakdown of our 100 patients. From this point forward, alternative Stata and/or Excel commands will be included in bold italics after the R commands, but outputs will not be shown (unless special features need explanation). As before, we can simply type the name of the variable using the dollar sign operator to print the vector of all 100 patient genders.

```
> df$Gender
[1] Male Female Male Female Female Male Male
[8] Female Female Female Male Female Female Female
[15] Female Male Male Male Female Female Female
[22] Female Male Male Male Male Female Male
[29] Female Male Female Female Male Female Female
[36] Male Female Female Female Male Male Male
[43] Female Female Male Female Female Female Male
[50] Female Female Female Female Female Female Female
[57] Female Female Female Male Male Male Male
[64] Female Male Female Female Male Female Female
[71] Male Male Male Female Female Female Male
[78] Male Male Male Male Female Female Male
[85] Male Female Female Female Male Female Female
[92] Male Male Male Male Male Female Female
[99] Female Male

Levels: Female Male
```

Stata: list gender

Gender is a categorical variable with two categories or "levels," in this case "male" and "female." A categorical variable is also known as a "factor" variable within R. This first step of describing a categorical variable is to simply count the number of instances of each category. We can do this using the table() function in R.

```
> table(df$Gender)
Female Male
56 44
```

Stata: **table gender**
Excel: **=countif (<array>, "Male") and =countif (<array>, "Female")**

The table() function shows us that we have 44 men and 56 women. To compute the sum of the men and women in the table, we can write sum(table(df$Gender)). This will return a value of 100. Using the sum that we have calculated, we can easily calculate the proportions of men and women in the sample.

```
> table(df$Gender)/(sum(table(df$Gender)))
Female Male
0.56 0.44
```

Stata: **tabulate gender**
Excel: **=[cell with countif total]/[sum(<array>)]**

R allows you to plot the aforementioned results graphically with a simple command (Figure 2.5).

Customizing the plot is relatively straightforward (Figure 2.6). The following code can be added to the plot() command to add a title, *x*- and *y*-axis labels, and *y*-axis limits.

```
> plot(df$Gender, main = "Gender Breakdown", ylab = "Number", xlab = "Gender", ylim = c(0,100))
```

Stata: **graph bar gender**
Excel: **<insert a bar graph with the two countif cells highlighted>**

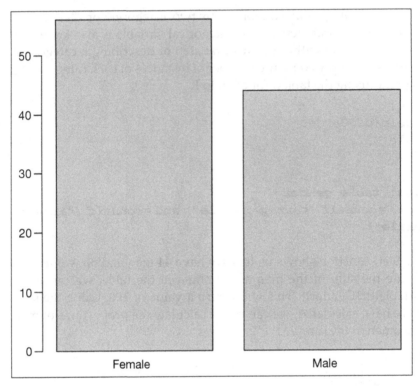

FIGURE 2.5
A bar plot of gender from R shows Female on the left and Male on the
right with the total number in the set for each given by the height of
the bar.

■ DESCRIBING AND GRAPHING CONTINUOUS VARIABLES

Now we will turn our attention to the variable df$Age, which, unlike
df$Gender, is continuous and stored as years. To describe a continuous
variable, we can calculate measures of central tendency and dispersion.
First, we will compute the mean age, the median age, and the different
percentiles. This is easily done in R with a simple line of code.

```
summary(df$Age)
Min. 1st Qu. Median Mean 3rd Qu. Max.  NA's
25.91 59.48  68.55  66.97 74.11  88.12 1
```

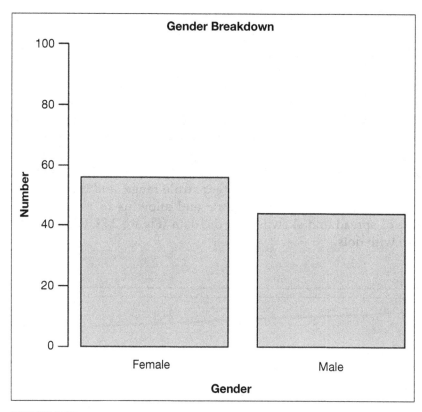

FIGURE 2.6
A customized bar plot from R showing labels for the graph and the axes, and with an axis adjustment to 100 units.

Stata: summarize gender, detail
Excel:=average(<array>),=median(<array>),=percentile
(<array>, %), =stdev(<array>)

R, like many statistical programs, has several different commands that can accomplish the same tasks. An alternative to the summary() function is the describe() function from the Hmisc library.

```
describe(df$Age)
df$Age
n missing unique Info Mean .05 .10 .25 .50 .75 .90 .95
```

```
99 1 95 1 66.97 49.27 50.87 59.48 68.55 74.11 80.61
83.83
lowest: 25.91 46.37 47.60 47.93 48.83, highest: 84.98
85.05 86.46 88.10 88.12
```

Having computed the summary statistics for df$Age, we now know how old our patients were on average at the time of surgery. However, computing summary statistics like these does not provide the full picture. To have a true understanding of the age distribution of the patients, we should explore them graphically. A box plot allows facile visualization of the median, the interquartile range, and the range of df$Age. Box plots are nonparametric and allow us to visualize the degree of spread and skewness in the data (Figure 2.7). Outliers are shown with dots.

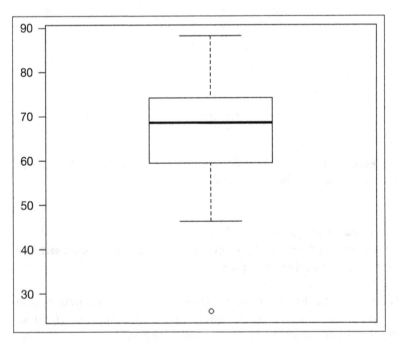

FIGURE 2.7
A box and whiskers plot produced by R is shown for age from our data set with the box representing the 25% (lower) and 75% (upper), the heavy black middle line representing the median, and the whiskers representing the limit of the outliers in either direction.

```
boxplot(df$Age)
```
Stata: graph box age

Another useful graphical tool is the histogram (Figure 2.8), which allows us to visualize the distribution of the variable df$Age. By visual inspection, we can ascertain whether the variable is normally distributed, skewed, or bimodal. In the succeeding section, we see that df$Age is approximately normally distributed, with some slight skewness to the left.

```
hist(df$Age)
```
Stata: histogram age, bin(50)

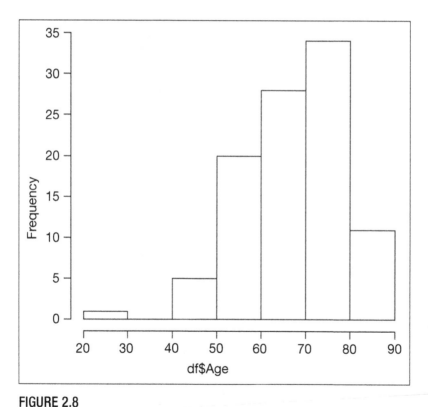

FIGURE 2.8
A histogram of age produced by R showing the distribution of values in the data set by the frequency at which they occur. Note that in Stata, the "bin" option determines the number of columns in the final histogram and ranges from 1 to 50.

We can smooth the histogram by instead creating a density plot. However, the density() function in R requires missing values to be removed from the vector prior to plotting. If we do not do that first, an error is generated:

```
> plot(density(df$Age))
Error in density.default(df$Age): 'x' contains missing
values
```

Stata: kdensity age

By using the na.omit() function, we can eliminate missing values prior to creating the density plot (Figure 2.9).

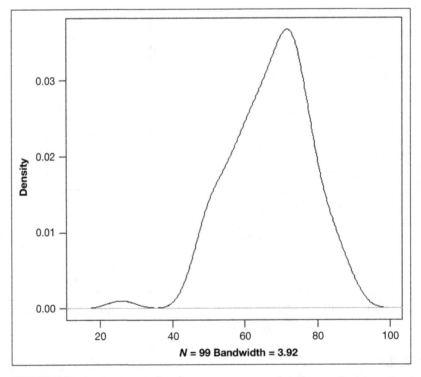

FIGURE 2.9
A kernel density plot of age produced by R, which shows a smoothed distribution of all variables as a percentage of the total data set.

```
plot(density(na.omit(df$Age)))
```

The box and whiskers plot, histogram, and smoothed density plots are simple yet powerful tools that allow for determination of a variety of statistical properties of the data by mere visual inspection. By visual inspection (if we know *n*), we can quickly make a determination of normality for small sets of cases. We may need to test normality formally or assume nonparametric distributions if the data appears skewed or has too few samples. In recent years, the violin plot has emerged as an alternative to these methods (Figure 2.10). A violin plot is essentially a combination of a box and whiskers plot and a smoothed histogram. The violin plot is one of the most powerful ways to visually explore data. R may be used to create violin plots via the vioplot()

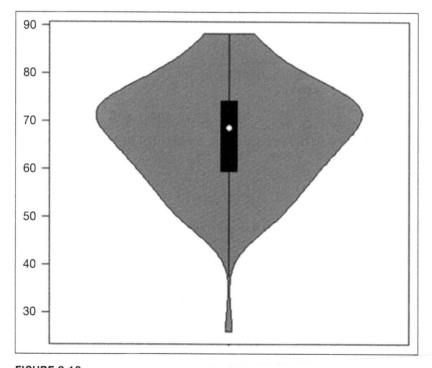

FIGURE 2.10
A violin plot of age produced in R shows a combination of the box and whisker plot with a smooth histogram. Note how it is clear that there are only a few outliers on the low side and a more abrupt end to the data on the high side.

library, which must be installed and loaded by the user. Again, missing values should be omitted.

```
install.packages("vioplot")
library(vioplot)
vioplot(na.omit(df$Age))
```

Measures of Dispersion

The standard deviation indicates the degree to which data points are spread out around the sample mean. Computing the standard deviation is simple in R. The sd() function can be modified to remove missing data by typing na.rm = T within its parentheses. We can see that the standard deviation of df$Age is approximately 11.

```
sd(df$Age, na.rm = T)
[1] 10.997
```

Stata: summarize age, detail
Excel: =stdev(<array>)

The standard error (i.e., the standard deviation of the mean) can also be easily computed in R. We recall from earlier that our mean age was:

```
mean(df$Age, na.rm = T)
[1] 66.96909
```

The standard error of the mean is defined as sd/√n. This can be computed in R as shown in the following. The length() function is employed to count the number of data points we have for df$Age.

```
sd(df$Age, na.rm = T)/sqrt(length(na.omit(df$Age)))
[1] 1.10524
```

Stata: summarize age, detail
Excel: =sterr(<array>)

We can also describe the skewness and kurtosis of continuous variables like df$Age. The e1071 package in R provides functions to perform these calculations and must be installed by the user.

```
install.packages("e1071")
library(e1071)
```

Skewness provides us with a way to measure the asymmetry of the probability distribution around a variable's mean. Recall from the previous section that, in our histogram of df$Age, we were able to visualize the left skewness in the variable. Using the e1071 library in R, we can quantify it with a number.

```
skewness(na.omit(df$Age))
[1] -0.5461206
```

Stata: summarize age, detail
Excel: =skew(<array>)

Kurtosis gives us a way to measure the "peakedness" of a variable's probability distribution. We can calculate it in R like so.

```
kurtosis(na.omit(df$Age))
[1] 0.6341401
```

Stata: summarize age, detail
Excel: =kurt(<array>)

The absolute moment can also be calculated in R using the moment() function.

```
moment(na.omit(df$Age))
[1] 66.96909
```

Let's summarize what we have covered so far. We started off by learning how to get our spreadsheet into R and Stata as well as reviewing it in Excel. Then we learned how to look at its contents from within all of them. We then looked at the user ID variable, a categorical or factor variable, and ensured that we had a unique ID for each patient. We then learned how to summarize the categorical variable df$Gender. We tabulated it, plotted it, and graphed it. Then we learned how to summarize, plot, and graph a continuous variable, df$Age. The next section details how to work with multiple variables at a time.

Dealing With Two Categorical Variables

We learned how to tabulate a categorical variable earlier. For example, df$Gender can be tabulated using the table() command in R.

```
table(df$Gender)
Female Male
56 44
```

Our data set also contains a categorical variable that indicates which side the surgical procedure was performed on: the left or the right. We can tabulate this as well.

```
table(df$Surgery_side)
Left Right
52 47
```

Stata: tabulate Surgery_side
Excel: =countif (<array>, "Left") and =countif (<array>, "Right")

We can perform a cross-tabulation of both variables simultaneously to learn more about the relationship (if any) between gender and side of surgery.[2] The code to do this is straightforward:

```
table(df$Gender, df$Surgery_side)
Left Right
Female 30 25
Male 22 22
```

Stata: table gender Surgery_side

We can create a bar graph (Figure 2.11) of the relative proportions of each of these categories like so:

```
plot(df$Gender, df$Surgery_side)
```

---

[2] If you wanted to know whether there was a statistically significant difference in the distribution between gender and surgery side, you could surround the code with chisq.test(). This will be covered in a later chapter.

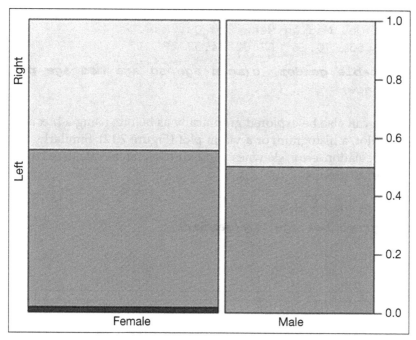

FIGURE 2.11
Stratified bar graph of gender by surgical side showing relative proportions of each. Note the small dark area at the bottom of the female graph, which denotes that the surgical side was not given in that patient.

Dealing With a Categorical Variable and a Continuous Variable

A categorical variable can also be related to a continuous variable. For example, we can explore the manner in which age varies with gender using R. We will use the same functions that we employed earlier in the chapter, this time programmed to stratify using the gender variable. As before, the describe() function can be used in place of the summary() function if desired.

```
# Summarize age stratified by gender
> tapply(df$Age, df$Gender, summary)
$Female
Min. 1st Qu. Median Mean 3rd Qu. Max.  NA's
25.91 60.58  68.01  66.93 74.62  88.10 1
```

```
$Male
Min. 1st Qu. Median Mean 3rd Qu. Max.
49.32 58.53   70.66   67.02 74.07   88.12
```

Stata: table gender, c(mean age sd age med age p25 age p75 age)

These data can also be explored graphically as before, using a box and whiskers plot, a histogram, or a violin plot (Figure 2.12). Similarly, the standard deviation, error, skewness, and kurtosis can be calculated over the categorical groups.

```
plot(df$Gender, df$Age)
```
Stata: graph box age, by(gender)

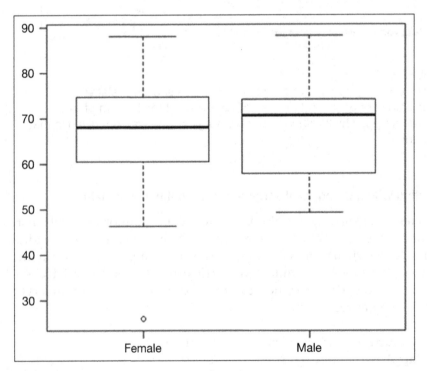

FIGURE 2.12
Stratified box and whiskers plot.

Confidence Intervals

This section describes the calculation of 95% confidence intervals.[3] To do this in R, we can use the CI() function from the Rmisc package. As before, we must install the package before using it for the first time, by typing install.packages("Rmisc"). Then we load it by typing library(Rmisc). The CI() function allows us to calculate the confidence interval for any vector of continuous data points. Let's try it for df$Age. As usual, since we have some missing data in this variable, we need to tell R to ignore them.

```
> CI(na.omit(df$Age))
upper mean lower
69.16240 66.96909 64.77578
```

By default, this command will give you the 95% confidence interval. But, if for some reason we want to calculate a different confidence interval, we can do so. Here is a way to calculate a 50% confidence interval.

```
> CI(na.omit(df$Age), ci = 0.50)
upper mean lower
67.71734 66.96909 66.22084
```

If we wanted to plot this result on a forest plot (also known as a confidence interval plot), we could use the forest() command from the package metaphor (which you need to install in the same manner that we did the other packages earlier in the chapter). It's a powerful command, and going into its intricate details is beyond the scope of this chapter, but for those who are interested, help can be found from within R by typing help(forest.default) after the package has been installed and loaded.

Dealing With Two Continuous Variables

We will now take a look at two continuous variables at once. For example, we can explore the relationship (if any) between patient age and tumor size in R by using the plot() command.

```
graph twoway scatter age tumor_size
plot(df$Age, df$Tumor_size)
```

---

[3] Inspecting the forest plot with its means and 95% confidence intervals is in essence a statistical hypothesis test asking if there is a significant difference between ages/ genders.

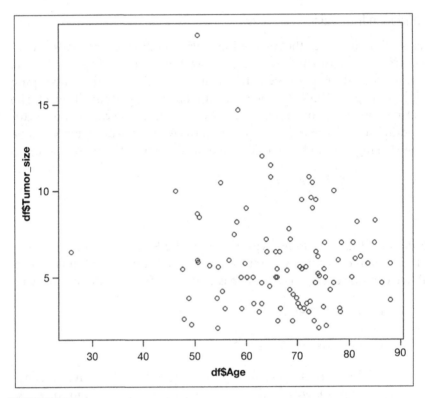

FIGURE 2.13
Plot of tumor size versus age.

As you can see in Figure 2.13, this code puts the tumor sizes on the *y*-axis and the corresponding patient ages on the *x*-axis. If we wanted to switch the axes, we could simply type plot(df$Tumor_size, df$Age). Before calculating a correlation coefficient between two continuous variables (which we will learn to do in Chapter 4), it's always a good idea to simply plot them for visual inspection, as previously mentioned.

■ SUMMARY AND CONCLUSIONS

That's it for our introduction to exploring our data with graphs and descriptive statistics. Our take-home lesson is that whenever approaching a data set, we should take a breath, slow down, and *simply look* at our data before getting fancy with statistical hypothesis tests. R, Stata, and Excel all offer ways to do this. Our advice would be to pick one, learn to use it well, and then use it often. Before diving into our next chapter on comparative statistics, let's try our hands on some self-study questions, as follows.

TAKE-HOME POINTS

- Understanding the format of your data prior to analysis, including the distribution, trends, and correlations, is key to meaningful analysis.

- Many tools are available to investigate individual variables as well as data sets, which allow for predictions about behavior in statistical analysis.

- Descriptive statistics of a data set are always required for a study even if the descriptive statistics are not reported in the final report.

QUESTIONS FOR SELF-STUDY

1. In our data set, some patients had their left kidneys removed, while others had their right kidneys removed. Some underwent laparoscopic surgeries while others underwent traditional open surgeries. Can you tabulate the number of individuals in each of the four groups (i.e., left/lap, left/open, right/lap, right/open) and then plot them graphically?

2. In our data set, patients had different tumor sizes. Can you calculate the mean and median tumor sizes, as well as find the range and interquartile range? Then, calculate the skewness of the tumor sizes and make a histogram. How do they compare?

3. Produce a table of the tumor stages of our patients, and then plot the data on a bar graph. Then, calculate descriptive summary statistics for patient age stratified by tumor stage.

ANSWERS TO QUESTIONS FOR SELF-STUDY

1. First, tabulate the results by typing table(df$Surgery_side, df$Surgery_type). Then, wrap this statement with the plot() command to create a graph: plot(table(df$Surgery_side, df$Surgery_type)).

2. After loading the Hmisc library, simply type describe(df$Tumor_size) to find the mean, median, and range of the tumor size variable. After loading the e1071 library, type skewness(df$Tumor_size) to calculate the skewness. The result indicates that we have a slight right skew. Does the histogram agree? Type hist(df$Tumor_size) to find out.

3. First, type table(df$Tumor_stage) to create a table. If you would like to view it in a column rather than a row, you can type as.matrix(table(df$Tumorstage)). To calculate age by tumor stage, use the tapply() function, like this: tapply(dfAge, dfTumor_stage, summary).

■ RECOMMENDED READING

R Core Team. R: A language and environment for statistical computing. R Foundation for Statistical Computing, Vienna, Austria, 2015. Available at https://www.R-project.org

StataCorp. *Stata Statistical Software: Release 14.* College Station, TX: StataCorp LP; 2015. Available at: http://www.cookbook-r.com/Statistical_analysis/Inter-rater_reliability

CHAPTER 3

Comparative Statistics

T. Rinda Soong
Danny A. Milner Jr.

■ INTRODUCTION

Let us consider groups of patients from various clinics of subspecialty medicine from the same hospital in the context of their clinical and laboratory data. Patients from the cardiac clinic versus patients from the renal clinic would likely have very different values for their ejection fraction, heart rate, C-reactive protein (CRP), creatinine, and blood urea nitrogen (BUN) such that we may even be able to guess beforehand which ones were "higher or lower on average" for each group. These preconceived thoughts are, in fact, our a priori hypotheses while the science of our approach would be to go and look at the values (to observe). Even after we do both things, however, the question remains: "Is the difference important?" In order to know that, we must apply a statistical test, the outcome of which is dependent on the form of the data, the distribution of the data, and the number of observations we have made. Comparative statistical testing is among the most common analyses employed to contrast outcomes under different conditions in medicine, including pathology studies. The first section of this chapter discusses the concepts related to sample inference, outlines the basic approach to testing, and summarizes the main assumptions and characteristics of common comparative tests used in research studies. With the use of selected examples, the next three sections illustrate the basic principles and considerations in performing comparative testing with numerical and categorical variables, interpreting test outcomes, and understanding

P values. Relationships among sample size, effect size, and power will also be briefly discussed and be revisited in the last chapter of the book.

■ WHAT IS STATISTICAL TESTING?

Sample Versus Population

Statistical analyses aid interpretation of research data in two ways: (a) by providing descriptive measures, which were discussed in Chapter 2, and (b) by making statistical inferences about population parameters and associations based on observations from a sample, which should be representative of the target population to maintain validity. Figure 3.1 shows a schematic diagram of the relationship between a target population and a research sample pertinent to statistical analyses.

In almost all cases, a representative sample is not a small replica of the target population with the exact same measures of distribution, unless the sample size is very large, hence warranting the need for statistical inference. Consider a crowded shopping mall on a Saturday in which we have three observers placed at three different locations as follows: at the main entrance near the parking lot, at the smaller entrance near public transportation, and outside the food court. If each of our observers asks 20 people the question "How did you get to the mall today?" we would expect that the first would be mostly driving, the second would be mostly public transportation, and the third would be a mixture. The third represents a more random sample and may give us better data about everyone in the mall while the first two samples are biased toward a specific type of transportation. This relationship between population and sample is perhaps best explained by the central limit theorem, which notes that, regardless of the shape of population distribution, the distribution of sample means will become closer and closer to the normal distribution in the population as the sample increases in size. Consider that if we asked everyone (let's assume 200 people) in the food court how they got to the mall, eventually we would be able to predict those by car and those by public transport because the sample would approach the means of the actual population.

Comparative statistics, which is the focus of this chapter, is one of the first steps to make inferences by quantitatively comparing samples

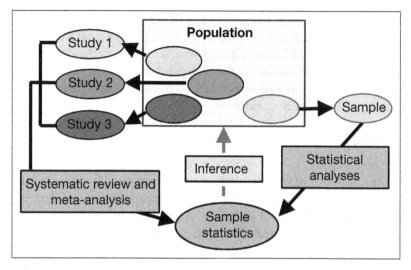

FIGURE 3.1
Schematic diagram showing how statistical analyses contribute to making inferences about population parameters based on a representative sample. Multiple studies can be done at different study sites or countries regarding the same population of interest. Due to variations in study designs, the findings may not be exactly the same across studies. One way to look at data from these different studies is to do a systematic review of their study designs and, if appropriate, combine the data using meta-analyses and obtain a weighted estimate for the parameter of interest in the target population.

For the purpose of this book we will focus on statistical methods that can be applied to one single study.

to decide whether observed differences in the sample data represent true differences in the target populations.

■ WHAT TESTS CAN WE USE?

Many tests are available for comparing measures of study samples (1,2). In general, statistical tests for comparison can be broadly classified based on their relevance to the data distribution and the data type of the dependent variables for comparison. In statistical analysis, we are interested in how the independent variables, i.e., the inputs or potential reasons for variations, are associated with the dependent variables, i.e., the characteristics of interest. For example, suppose we hypothesize that the tumor size of colon cancer is different between the left and right colon and then set up a study to compare tumor size based on the tumor location (left vs. right). The tumor size would be the dependent variable and tumor location would be the independent variable. For typical comparisons, there is only one dependent variable at a time while there may be many independent variables.

■ TEST SELECTION

Different tests apply to different study designs, data types, data distributions, number of independent variables involved in the comparison, as well as sample measures of interest. Appropriate test selection is crucial for correct statistical inference. A simplified flowchart on test selection is proposed in Figure 3.2, with summary of the characteristics of the most common tests reported in research literature listed in Tables 3.1 and 3.2. Note that many tests have a parametric and a nonparametric version in this table; however, that is not always the case.

(text continues on page 48)

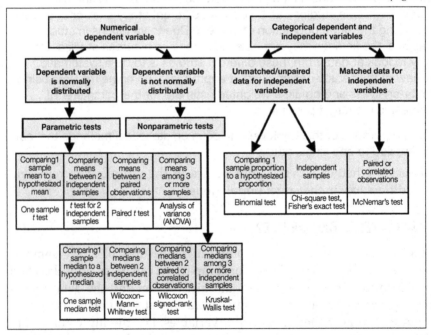

FIGURE 3.2
Common comparative tests based on data type, study design, and data distribution.

TABLE 3.1
Common Statistical Tests for Comparing Samples With a Numerical Dependent Variable

		NUMERICAL DEPENDENT VARIABLE			
PARAMETRIC TESTS	NUMBER OF GROUP(S) FOR COMPARISON	ASSUMPTIONS	NULL HYPOTHESIS	TEST STATISTIC	NON-PARAMETRIC COUNTERPART
One-sample *t* test (rarely used in pathology studies)	1	• The dependent variable is a numerical variable. • The dependent variable is normally distributed. • Observations are independent of each other (data are not correlated).	The mean in the population is the same as the hypothesized mean.	t-statistic	One-sample median test (rarely used in pathology studies)

(continued)

TABLE 3.1
Common Statistical Tests for Comparing Samples With a Numerical Dependent Variable (*continued*)

		NUMERICAL DEPENDENT VARIABLE			
PARAMETRIC TESTS	NUMBER OF GROUP(S) FOR COMPARISON	ASSUMPTIONS	NULL HYPOTHESIS	TEST STATISTIC	NON-PARAMETRIC COUNTERPART
Two-independent-sample *t* test (*t* test/ Student's *t* test)	2	• The dependent variable is a numerical variable. • The dependent variable is normally distributed in both groups. • Observations are independent of each other (data are not correlated). • For comparison between two groups: The population variances are equal to each other.	The means are the same in the two populations in comparison.	t-statistic	Wilcoxon–Mann–Whitney test (Mann–Whitney U test, Wilcoxon rank-sum test)

(continued)

TABLE 3.1
Common Statistical Tests for Comparing Samples With a Numerical Dependent Variable (*continued*)

PARAMETRIC TESTS	NUMBER OF GROUP(S) FOR COMPARISON	NUMERICAL DEPENDENT VARIABLE			
		ASSUMPTIONS	NULL HYPOTHESIS	TEST STATISTIC	NON-PARAMETRIC COUNTERPART
Paired *t* test (paired Student's *t* test)	2	• The dependent variable is a numerical variable. • The differences from each data pair are normally distributed. • Observations are paired.	The means of the correlated/ matched populations are not different from each other.	t-statistic	Wilcoxon signed-rank test
One-way ANOVA	3 or more	• The dependent variable is a numerical variable. • The dependent variable is normally distributed in each of the groups. • Observations within a group are independent of each other. • The within-group variance is the same across all groups.	The mean is the same across all the sampled populations.	F-statistic	Kruskal–Wallis test

ANOVA, Analysis of variance

TABLE 3.2
Common Statistical Tests for Comparing Samples With a Categorical Dependent Variable

TESTS	NUMBER OF GROUP(S) FOR COMPARISON	CATEGORICAL VARIABLE		
		ASSUMPTIONS AND APPROPRIATE DATA	NULL HYPOTHESIS	TEST STATISTIC
Binomial test	1	• The variable is dichotomous. • Observations are independent of each other. • The test is nonparametric.	The proportion is the same as the hypothesized value.	Z-score when normal approximation is justified; otherwise it is an exact test of probability.
Chi-square goodness-of-fit test	2	• The variable is categorical. • Observations are independent of each other (data are not correlated). • The test compares observed to expected frequencies in each category under the assumption of no association to compute a χ^2 statistic, which follows a χ^2 distribution	There is no association between the two categorical variables.	χ^2 test statistic

(continued)

TABLE 3.2
Common Statistical Tests for Comparing Samples With a Categorical Dependent Variable (*continued*)

		CATEGORICAL VARIABLE		
TESTS	NUMBER OF GROUP(S) FOR COMPARISON	ASSUMPTIONS AND APPROPRIATE DATA	NULL HYPOTHESIS	TEST STATISTIC
McNemar's test	2	<ul><li>The variable is categorical.</li><li>Observations are paired/ matched.</li><li>If number of discordant pairs is < 20, a test based on exact binomial probabilities is needed.</li></ul>	The marginal probabilities of each of the outcomes are the same.	χ^2 test statistic

For example, a one-way analysis of variance (ANOVA) is described but there can also be a two-way ANOVA (a very common test in experimental literature), which, in fact, does not have a nonparametric equivalent. Thus, adequate sample size and evaluation for test assumptions for two-way ANOVA are key.

The first two steps in test selection are to decide what data type and distribution are observed with the variables of interest.

■ TYPES OF VARIABLES GOVERN TEST SELECTION

The type of a data variable depends on the nature of the measurement and is subject to a researcher's judgment based on the study context. For the purpose of statistical comparative testing, the key distinction is between categorical and numerical variables.

Categorical variables: These are qualitative variables that are collected or described in categories. Such a variable is ordinal if the categories can be logically and meaningfully ordered, e.g., histologic grade (well, moderately, and poorly differentiated), tumor stage (I, II, III, etc.). It is important to note that these ordinal categories go in a specific order, but there is not necessarily a quantitative relationship between them that is easily measured. Otherwise, the categorical variable is described as unordered or nominal. Some examples include gender or ethnicity. In pathology, we may have a categorical classification that appears mixed but the analysis is still done in only one way. For example, if we are cataloging all tumors of the uterus and classify stromal masses as leiomyoma, leiomyosarcoma, endometrial stromal tumor, or endometrial adenocarcinoma, there may exist some quantitative or biological relationship between leiomyoma and leiomyosarcoma but, in this variable, we analyze as if these are unordered categories, meaning that all categories have an equal, independent chance of assignment to a patient.

Numerical variables: These are variables that are either described with a discrete set of values (e.g., count data such as number of positive Pap smears in a woman in the past or number of mitoses in 20 high-power fields), or take on a continuum of values (e.g., age or gene expression level). This will be further discussed in the chapter on Poisson count data (Chapter 6).

The difference between ordinal and nominal categorical variables, or the distinction between discrete and continuous numerical variables, does not affect the choice of comparative tests. Their recognitions, however, would be important in further statistical analyses, for example, selection of statistical models for estimating effect size, which will be discussed in Chapter 5 and Chapter 6.

As one may suspect, overlap between data types is possible. For example, numerical variables, such as age or Ki67 immunostaining index in image analysis, can be described in meaningful categories, in which case comparison with a test for categorical variables should be used. Consider that if all ages are recorded for a group of 200 patients with World Health Organization (WHO)-staged glomerulonephritis, we can categorize age as "less than 45 years of age" and "greater than or equal to 45 years of age," which reduces our very granular individual age data to a simple binary (yes/no) categorical variable. Categorizing a numerical variable inherently results in loss of information on data variation, as values in the same category would be treated the same. As such, categorization should not be made solely on arbitrary or convenience grounds, but should be considered based on the research question, cutoffs relevant to clinical practice, as well as data distribution such as presence of multimodal distribution in observed data (as visualized on a histogram in Chapter 2).

The distinction between categorical and numerical variables may not always be straightforward. Ordinal variables, particularly those with limited numbers on a scale (e.g., 0, 1+, 2+, 3+ in immunohistochemical (IHC) studies or histologic scores for breast cancer) may raise potential confusion in analysis. This is partly because such data are to a certain extent quantitative, and partly because the quantitative differences between the numbers/categories of many of these entities are challenging to specify in pathology studies. Consider having three different pathologists (who have never met) score an IHC stain for estrogen receptor versus having a computer analyze images from the same cases. Unless prior consensus has been reached, pathologists' review is subject to individual judgement call and it is easy to understand how one pathologist's 2+ may be another pathologist's 3+ due to different levels of experience or opinions. Digital image analysis via a computer, on the other hand, may help yield objective numerical IHC scores according to empirical data on predefined parameters. Depending on the scope of parameters used for data collection, however, the classification "scale" yielded by a computer may be less subtle than the pathologist's eye is capable of splitting. While methods of analysis vary by research settings and there is often no strict universal way to describe a particular variable across studies, it is reasonable to describe these data as categorical variables while we cannot make the assumption that the differences between values are quantifiable, or at least not uniformly quantifiable. Models have been proposed to assign distances between categories via optimal scaling to analyze them as numerical variables, mostly in the setting of regression and multivariate analyses and in sociologic or psychologic studies (3,4). Caution should be exercised so as to avoid jumping at a naive assumption on ordinal data as being numerical variables with quantifiable differences between values, and insensibly applying methods, e.g., comparison of means and general linear regression, to these data without justification or data checking. For example, consider expression profile data (often given as fold change, which is relative but quantitative) in comparison to IHC stain for the protein produced by the gene (scored 0, 1+, 2+, 3+, 4+) where our data show that a twofold increase in expression results in a higher response rate to a given chemotherapy. We might assume that 2+ versus 4+ is an equivalent change to twofold overexpression; however, this is simply not true a priori and such supposition could greatly damage any study resulting in false data interpretation.

■ PARAMETRIC VERSUS NONPARAMETRIC TESTS

Examination of data distribution of a *numerical* dependent variable of interest is important as it helps us to decide whether assumptions of a particular test on data distribution are met. Comparative statistical tests can be classified based on that regard into parametric tests and nonparametric tests, a summary of which is given in Tables 3.1 and 3.2.

Parametric tests are applicable to those data for which distribution assumptions can be made on the dependent variable of interest, the most common of which is an assumption of normal distribution.

Nonparametric tests are used when we do not have good evidence or prior data to support a data distribution assumption. These tests are suitable for data with a skewed distribution, with a discrete scale, or already in a form of ranks. They have the advantage of relaxing distribution assumptions. Applying a nonparametric test, like Wilcoxon–Mann–Whitney test, to comparison with data that are known to be normally distributed would lead to reduction of power to detect a difference. The reason is that nonparametric tests work by assigning ranks to data and comparing the ranks, without accounting for the actual size difference between sample values. To view it the other way, a parametric test, such as *t* test, is sensitive to outliers and the test outcome can easily be influenced by presence of just one or two extreme outliers. In contrast, presence of a couple of outliers does not alter the test results of its nonparametric counterpart, Wilcoxon–Mann–Whitney test, because the rank scheme remains unchanged. To consider this practically, assume we have a collection of patients ($n = 10,000$) from the emergency room of a large tertiary care hospital and we want to compare the body temperatures of subgroups with different clinical characteristics. For parametric tests, their actual temperatures on scale are evaluated. For nonparametric tests, the patients are ranked from 1 to 10,000 from the lowest to the highest temperatures. Since the sample size is fairly large, the distribution of temperatures of the whole cohort would be roughly Gaussian (or normal) and the mean and median for the total patient group would be minimally affected by removing any one patient. If we look at only a subset ($n = 500$) who presented with any sign of infection (some with fever and some without), we would expect there to be a skew of high temperatures and the mean would be affected by excluding (or including) patients with high fever. However, the ranks (1 through 500) will not be affected by removing one or more patients. Note that as the number of samples decreases in a set, the effect on the mean (compared in t-test) becomes more unstable while the effect on the median (compared in Wilcoxon–Mann–Whitney test) has little change.

◼ HYPOTHESIS TESTING

Hypothesis testing is the conceptual foundation of comparative statistics and statistical modeling. In general, four steps are involved in performing a statistical test, the first three of which should ideally be done during study design and not after the data are collected to avoid the trap of data fishing or P-hacking.

Before we do a statistical test, we need to: (a) identify the null and alternative hypotheses; (b) decide on a test that is appropriate for the data type, data distribution, and study design; (c) determine a priori the probability threshold below which the null hypothesis is rejected; and (d) perform the test, and interpret the P value associated with the test statistic and conclude whether the test result is statistically significant.

The aforementioned steps introduce a number of important statistical concepts. We will go over their definitions and will discuss them in the context of examples in the next three sections:

Hypothesis: Every statistical test is based on a null hypothesis (H_0) and an alternative hypothesis (H_A). In general, the null hypothesis states that there is no difference in the *populations* in comparison in terms of the measure in question, and the alternative hypothesis states the otherwise. The respective null hypotheses for the different tests are listed in Tables 3.1 and 3.2. Suppose we have been reading patient charts from an arthritis clinic in a group of people with an average age of 63 years, and we want to examine whether replaced joints show chronic synovitis dependent on age. A null hypothesis from this data might be that there is no relationship between age and chronic synovitis. An alternative hypothesis from this data might be that there is a directly proportional relationship between age and the presence of chronic synovitis. It is most important to note, however, that another alternative hypothesis is that there is an inverse relationship between age and chronic synovitis. We must, at this point, test these hypotheses to move forward.

Table 3.3 shows the relationship of hypothesis testing with type I and type II errors.

Type I error (α) is the probability of rejecting a null hypothesis when it is actually true. In practice, we generally apply a conventional $\alpha = 0.05$, meaning that we expect a 5% chance of making a false positive inference. Violations of assumptions of comparative tests would result in a greater type I error rate than we commit to prior to testing. Note that α is not a P value but rather the threshold value with which a calculated P value will be compared.

Type II error (β) is the probability of missing a difference or association (false negative error) in a study.

TABLE 3.3
Type I and Type II Errors in Relation to Hypothesis Testing

	TRUE STATE OF NULL HYPOTHESIS	
STATISTICAL DECISION	H_0 TRUE (EXAMPLE: THERE IS NO DIFFERENCE IN MEANS BETWEEN THE TWO POPULATIONS)	H_0 FALSE (EXAMPLE: THERE IS A DIFFERENCE IN MEANS BETWEEN THE TWO POPULATIONS)
Reject H_0	**Type I error (α)**	Correct
Do not reject H_0	Correct	**Type II error (β)**

Power (1–β) is the probability of correctly rejecting a false null hypothesis if the alternative hypothesis is true. In other words, it refers to the power of the study to detect a hypothesized effect size if the effect truly exists in the population. In general, 80% power (or $\beta = 0.20$) is standard for most studies. Power (and thus β) is affected by sample size, while α is arbitrarily set and the resulting P value (see the following section) is affected by sample size.

P value is defined as the probability of obtaining the observed or a more extreme result if the null hypothesis is true. It should be noted that the P value is a conditional probability based on the null hypothesis. When the P value is less than α, the null hypothesis can be rejected and the test result is deemed statistically significant in that experiment.

With these general definitions in mind, let's move on to see how these work in the context of examples.

■ EXAMPLE: BLOOD MICRORNA EXPRESSION IN RELATION TO BREAST CANCER RECURRENCE

MicroRNAs (miRNAs) in blood have been suggested to be prognostic factors for metastatic breast cancer (5). Consider the following study.

Hypothetical Study

A research group showed in mouse models that the ratio of miR-101/miR-25 (miR ratio) is associated with development of metastatic disease. A pilot study was performed to investigate whether the association may exist in humans. Blood samples were pulled from a biorepository for breast cancer patients who underwent lumpectomy and axillary lymph node dissection. Blood samples were extracted from patients who did not have lymph node metastasis ($n = 15$) and from patients who had lymph node metastasis ($n = 15$). The blood samples collected were from baseline visit before lumpectomy. Reverse transcription polymerase chain reaction (RT-PCR)-based assays were used to assess miR-101 and miR-25 levels in the blood samples. Data outputs given in the following are based on a hypothetical data set (**see online materials; available at www.demosmedical.com/pathology-data-sets**). The analyses were performed with Stata using two different commands: (a) **sort Metastasis** and (b) **by Metastasis: summarize miR_ratio**. Figure 3.3 shows a brief data summary and Figure 3.4 illustrates the box plots of miR ratios in patients with and without metastasis from the command **graph box miR_ratio, over (Metastasis)**. Our observation (the science) is that, by

```
. sort  Metastasis

. by Metastasis: summarize miR_ratio


-> Metastasis = without lymph node metastasis
     variable |      obs       Mean    std. Dev.         Min        Max
    miR_ratio |       15       .318     .1508168         .05        .61


-> Metastasis = with lymph node metastasis
     variable |      obs       Mean    std. Dev.         Min        Max
    miR_ratio |       15       .628     .1658399          .3        .95
```

FIGURE 3.3
Means and standard deviations of miR ratios in patients with and without
lymph node metastasis.

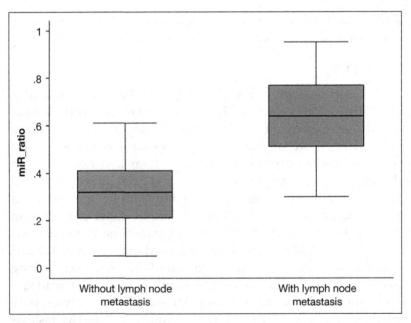

FIGURE 3.4
Box plots of miR ratios in patients with and without axillary lymph node
metastasis.

eye, it appears that the median and mean miR ratios are higher among those with lymph node metastasis, but is the difference statistically significant and what test can we do to check that?

What test should we do? The dependent variable, miR ratio, is numerical. The next question we should ask is whether a parametric or a nonparametric test should be used for comparison, which calls for evaluation for data normality. There are several ways to test for normality, including graphical methods, such as a histogram, Q-Q plot, P-P plot, box plot; or numerical tests, such as Shapiro-Wilk test, Shapiro-Francia test, Kolmogorov-Smirnov test; or tests for skewness/kurtosis may also be used for testing the hypothesis of normality. Figure 3.5 shows a normal Q-Q plot, which compares by quantiles the observed data distribution of the miR ratios with a theoretical normal distribution. This is obtained by the command **qnorm miR_ratio**. If all the data points fall along the straight line, then there is a perfect fit with normal distribution. Any systematic deviation from the straight line would indicate that the data are from distributions other than normal. By eyeballing it seems that the data in both groups in our study are roughly following a normal distribution. Box plots show that the median (the line in the middle of the box) is close to the center of the box and there is no outlier (Figure 3.4), suggesting there is no skew in the data distribution. The mean and the median (50% percentile) should be the same

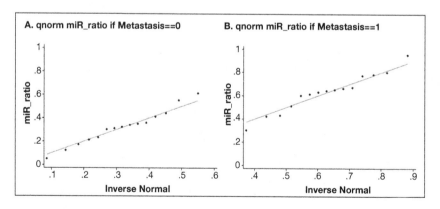

FIGURE 3.5
Q-Q plots of miR ratios. (A) Q-Q plot of miR ratios of patients without lymph node metastasis. (B) Q-Q plot of miR ratios of patients with lymph node metastasis.

or very close to each other in a normal distribution. Shapiro-Wilk test performed in this study sample shows that the hypothesis of normality cannot be rejected as probability $>z$ is > 0.05 (Figure 3.6), supporting the observation of a normal distribution (command **swilk miR_ratio**). Given these findings, it is reasonable to perform a two independent sample t test to compare the mean miR ratios between the two groups.

How do we interpret the t test and P value? The null hypothesis is that the mean miR ratios are the same between patients with and without lymph node metastases. The α is set at 0.05 for this

```
. by Metastasis: swilk miR_ratio

-> Metastasis = without lymph node metastasis

                    Shapiro-wilk W test for normal data

    Variable |    Obs        W         V         z      Prob>z

    miR_ratio |    15     0.98058    0.377    -1.932    0.97332

-> Metastasis = with lymph node metastasis

                    Shapiro-wilk W test for normal data

    Variable |    Obs        W         V         z      Prob>z

    miR_ratio |    15     0.97026    0.577    -1.089    0.86187
```

FIGURE 3.6
Shapiro-Wilk test for normality of miR ratio data.

```
. ttest miR_ratio, by (Metastasis) unequal

Two-sample t test with unequal variances

    Group |   Obs      Mean     std. Err.   std. Dev.   [95% Conf. Interval]

with met |    15      .628     .0428197    .1658399    .536161    .719839
  No met |    15      .318     .0389407    .1508168    .2344804   .4015196

combined |    30      .473     .0404604    .2216109    .3902491   .5557509

    diff |             .31      .0578784                .1913937   .4286063

    diff = mean(with met) - mean(No met)                      t =   5.3561
Ho: diff = 0                        Satterthwaite's degrees of freedom =  27.7513

    Ha: diff < 0                    Ha: diff != 0                   Ha: diff > 0
 Pr(T < t) = 1.0000          Pr(|T| > |t|) = 0.0000          Pr(T > t) = 0.0000
```

FIGURE 3.7
Two independent samples t test on miR ratios in patients with nodal metastasis versus those without nodal metastasis.

comparison. Figure 3.7 illustrates the *t* test output given by the command **ttest miR_ratio, by (Metastasis) unequal**. The observed difference of miR ratios is 0.31. The difference of miR ratios (95% CI for the estimate in the populations: 0.19–0.43) is statistically significant ($P < .001$) in the two-sided test. This is supported by the P values (".0000" which we interpret as $P < .001$) associated with the alternative hypotheses ("Ha") that the difference of miR ratios is not equal to zero ("diff ! = 0") or the difference is greater than zero ("diff > 0").

What does the P value mean exactly? The P value is *not* the probability that the null hypothesis is true, *nor* is it the probability that the observed difference is merely due to chance. In this example, the P value gives the probability ($< 0.1\%$) of getting a t-statistic at or more extreme than the observed value (5.35) (Figure 3.7), under the null hypothesis that the mean miR ratios are the same in the two patient populations being compared. The concept of P value can be demonstrated with a thought experiment (Figure 3.8). Imagine we have the resources to draw infinite repeated samples from the two patient populations of interest. Each sample will have its own mean miR ratio. We then calculate the differences between the mean miR ratios with each sample drawn from these two patient populations. If the null hypothesis is true, that is, there is no difference in miR ratio means between these two populations, the differences of these miR ratio means will follow a normal distribution around "0," as illustrated in Figure 3.8B. The gray shaded area represents graphically the threshold percentage for statistical significance, that is α. The black shaded area represents the probability, that is, the P value ($< 0.1\%$ in this example) of repeated samples that yield the same or greater test statistic if the null hypothesis is true. Since $\alpha = 0.05$ in this example, a P value of $< .05$ allows us to reject the null hypothesis.

CAVEATS

Two-sided versus one-sided hypothesis testing: In this example, we are performing a two-sided test, that is, testing the hypothesis in both directions, which apply to most studies. A one-sided test is much less common and should be done only when there is strong prior data indicating a particular direction of the effect of interest. Since the one-sided test is designed to test the association in only one direction, it results in more power to detect an effect and a lower P value, which should not

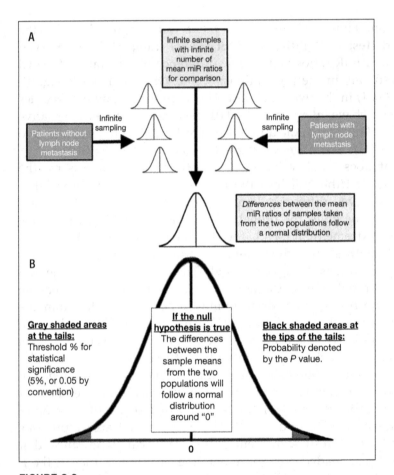

FIGURE 3.8

Schematic diagram of a thought experiment exemplifying the concept of P value. (A) Infinite repeated samples are drawn from the two populations of interest. Each sample will yield its own mean miR ratio. (B) If the null hypothesis is true, the differences of these miR ratio means from the two populations will center around "0" in a normal distribution. The gray shaded area represents graphically the threshold percentage for statistical significance, i.e., α. The black shaded area represents the probability, i.e., the P value, of repeated samples that yield the same or greater observed difference if the null hypothesis is true.

be the sole motivation for performing a one-sided test. To illustrate this, consider that we have two patient groups who are randomly assigned to receive either a placebo (cellulose pill) or an oral hypoglycemic, which has its maximal effect at 2 hours after ingestion. We may assume that the placebo group will have higher glucose than the drug group; however, in reality, either group could have a higher glucose biologically. Thus, a two-sided test is required to ensure statistical rigor. Only rarely are one-sided tests allowed (see Chapter 6).

Equal versus unequal variance: As stated in Table 3.1, one of the assumptions for a two-sample *t* test is equal variance in the samples. In most cases the *t* test is very robust with respect to this assumption, meaning that the type I error rate is not seriously affected by violation of this assumption. However, when sample sizes are not equal, the type I error rate can increase substantially. This problem can be solved by doing a version of *t* test for unequal variances, aka the Welch's variant of *t* test, which is readily available in most statistical packages. As an example, consider a population of pediatric patients who present with coma, peripheral blood parasitemia for malaria, and no other cause of coma that can be determined (i.e., these children clinically have cerebral malaria) versus controls who may not have coma or parasitemia, or may have another cause of coma. In the former group, we would expect any variable to have a variance specific to cerebral malaria, whereas in the control group, any variable will likely have a much higher variance due to inherent heterogeneity in the patient population. This can be tested for any given variable by evaluating the standard deviation and/or variance directly by inspection.

Normal versus nonnormal data distribution: The assumption of normality for *t* test can be relaxed with larger samples because the difference of the means converges to a normal distribution when sample size increases. With small samples, the effect of violation of the normality assumption on the type I error rate is usually conservative, meaning that it becomes more likely for us to accept the null hypothesis when real difference exists. In the setting of a two-sample comparison, if group sizes differ greatly, or if one or both of the groups' data are not normally distributed, then it is inappropriate to apply the *t* test. One way to tackle this problem is to normalize the data by transforming it (Figure 3.9), which is useful in settings when one plans to further analyze the transformed data with a linear model. Another option is to do a nonparametric test, such as Wilcoxon–Mann–Whitney test.

Correlated versus uncorrelated samples: Correlation between samples arises when data are matched. Even a small amount of correlation

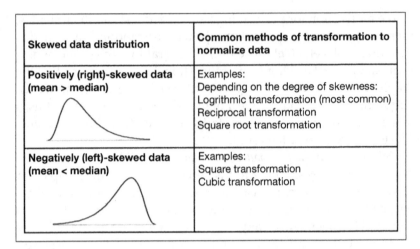

Skewed data distribution	Common methods of transformation to normalize data
Positively (right)-skewed data (mean > median)	Examples: Depending on the degree of skewness: Logrithmic transformation (most common) Reciprocal transformation Square root transformation
Negatively (left)-skewed data (mean < median)	Examples: Square transformation Cubic transformation

FIGURE 3.9
Common methods of transformation for data with skewed distribution.

can make the test difficult to interpret due to its impact on the type I error rate. If means or medians need to be compared between matched samples, a paired t test (parametric) or a Wilcoxon signed-rank test (nonparametric) should be considered for testing. A classic example in pathology is a biopsy versus a resection (with or without treatment) where the histological samples are biologically identical to each other and should be compared using paired tests.

Presence of outliers: Before doing the test, it is important to look at the data distribution and assess for presence of outliers, as they can significantly skew the data distribution and test statistics. Data points which deviate too much from other observations may potentially suggest that they are intrinsically different from the rest of the population, for example, disease arising via a different mechanism or error in sample measurement/collection, necessitating review of the data in correlation with other variables in the study. Repeat measurement may also be warranted in appropriate settings. Simple exclusion of outliers from study analysis without justification and data review is inappropriate and should not be done to produce a "clean" or statistically significant result. A great example of outliers are peripheral blood biomarkers that are quantified for patients but do not have an upper limit (either through dynamic range or by dilutional testing). Consider prostate-specific antigen (PSA) in a group of men where one third are normal, one third have benign prostatic hypertrophy (BPH), and one third have a range of prostate cancer stages. We would fully expect that the prostate cancer patients have PSAs in the hundreds and maybe a rare one in the thousands. However, 66% of our data will be in the less than 20 range. These cancer patients' data technically may look like an outlier; however, there is a biological explanation and we must adjust our statistical testing to account for that.

■ EXAMPLE: SERUM CREATININE LEVELS IN CHRONIC KIDNEY DISEASE

UBIAD1, an intracellular cholesterol regulator, has been suggested to play a role in vascular cell calcification (6). Consider the following study.

Hypothetical Study

A CRISPR/CAS9 tool was developed to replace the UBIAD1 gene with an inactive form of the protein. It was hypothesized that the gene product may help reduce calcification and improve kidney function. Control and 5/6Nx rat models of chronic kidney disease (CKD) were used in the study to test this hypothesis. 5/6Nx rats develop CKD including vascular calcifications and disease was monitored using peripheral blood measure of creatinine prior to euthanasia. Figure 3.10 shows the creatinine levels of the control rats ($n = 10$), 5/6Nx rats with active UBIAD1 gene (NxBIAD1a; $n = 10$), and 5/6Nx rats with inactive UBIAD1 gene (NxBIAD1i; $n = 10$) based on a hypothetical data set. What test should we do to compare the creatinine levels by the rat groups? Figure 3.10 shows

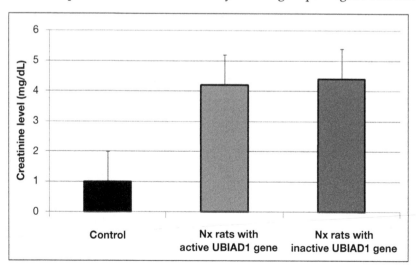

FIGURE 3.10
Bar chart showing creatinine levels (mean ± SD) across rat groups.

the creatinine levels in a bar chart. The "error" bars on the chart represent the standard deviations, aka the spread, of the measurements in the samples. In such context, do not be tempted to show the standard errors of the means (SEMs) (which are estimated measures of the population) because they are smaller and look better on the chart (7). Exploratory analysis suggests that the data points roughly follow a normal distribution (same steps as shown in earlier example of blood microRNAs; data not shown); the standard deviations as well as the variances are roughly equal across the three rat groups as suggested by the error bars. The observations are not correlated, meaning the samples are not matched and each measurement is independent. Thus, one-way ANOVA would be a good choice of test in this setting as we want to look at the mean of a continuous variable in more than two groups.

How should we interpret the test? Figure 3.11 shows the test output of the one-way ANOVA give by the command **oneway Creatinine Rat_group, tabulate (see online materials; available at www.demosmedical .com/pathology-data-sets)**. The P value for the Bartlett's test for equal variance is greater than 0.05, hence we cannot reject the null hypothesis of equal variance across the three groups. The F-test in one-way ANOVA assesses the null hypothesis that the mean value of creatinine is the same across the three rat populations, against the alternative hypothesis that the means differ in at least two of the populations. In Figure 3.11, the F-test ($P < .001$) suggests that at least two groups differ by their mean creatinine levels. Based on Figure 3.10, we can readily suspect that the

```
. oneway  Creatinine Rat_group, tabulate
```

Rat_group	Summary of Creatinine Mean	Std. Dev.	Freq.
control	.97464815	.20531289	10
NxBIAD1a	4.3743441	.19402332	10
NxBIAD1i	4.4125812	.22841003	10
Total	3.2538578	1.6517179	30

Source	Analysis of variance SS	df	MS	F	Prob > F
Between groups	77.9292617	2	38.9646308	885.76	0.0000
Within groups	1.18772615	27	.043989857		
Total	79.1169878	29	2.72817199		

```
Bartlett's test for equal variances:  chi2(2) =  0.2387  Prob>chi2 = 0.887
```

FIGURE 3.11
ANOVA output on comparison of creatinine levels across three rat groups.

difference exists between 5/6Nx rats and control rats, and the difference in creatinine levels likely has no association with inactivation of the UBIAD1 gene. We can perform multiple pairwise testing to check for the statistical significance of the difference.

How do we interpret the P value in multiple hypothesis testing? It is important to note that the actual type I error rate would be greater than α if we keep our a priori α at 0.05 with multiple testing. In this particular study example:

Probability (at least one significant result due to random chance) =
1 – Probability (no significant result) =
$1 - (1 - 0.05)^3 = 0.14$

In other words, the actual type I error rate would be raised to 14% if we keep our a priori α at 0.05 when we perform the three pairwise tests. The α therefore needs to be adjusted for correct interpretation of P value. With a small number of tests, the most common method used is perhaps the Bonferroni correction, via which each P value is compared with a corrected significance level: 0.05/(number of planned pairwise comparisons). In the Stata outputs, the results are presented as a matrix (Figure 3.12) and given by the command [**oneway Creatinine Rat_group, bonferroni**]. The first entry, 3.3997, represents the difference between the mean creatinine levels from the control rats and NxBIAD1i rats. Underneath that number is reported "0.000." This is

```
. oneway  Creatinine Rat_group, bonferroni

                        Analysis of Variance
      Source            SS           df      MS           F       Prob > F

Between groups     77.9292617         2   38.9646308    885.76    0.0000
 within groups      1.18772615       27   .043989857

     Total         79.1169878        29   2.72817199

Bartlett's test for equal variances:   chi2(2) =   0.2387  Prob>chi2 = 0.887

                      Comparison of Creatinine by Rat_group
                                  (Bonferroni)
Row Mean-|
Col Mean |     control    NxIBAIDa

NxBIAD1a |     3.3997
         |     0.000

NxBIAD1i |     3.43793     .038237
         |     0.000        1.000
```

FIGURE 3.12
Pairwise testing of creatinine levels with Bonferroni correction.

the Bonferroni-adjusted significance of the difference. In this example, the differences are statistically significant between the control and NxBIAD1a rats, and between the control and NxBIAD1i rats. Had the observed differences been not that big, the conclusion would have been vulnerable to an erroneous null if no correction is done on α before doing the test. The concept of α adjustment applies not just to ANOVA but to all settings of multiple hypothesis testing, such as correlations of gene expression levels in large-scale studies (8).

CAVEATS

Other methods to correct for multiple hypothesis testing: Methods of correction are roughly of two classes: (a) correction of the familywise error rate (FWER) and (b) correction of the false discovery rate (FDR), which can be easily performed in most statistical packages. Bonferroni correction is one of the simplest FWER methods that control the probability of committing even one type I error across all. The disadvantage is that the method is very conservative and significantly reduces power as the number of tests increases. Other FWER methods, e.g., Holm's and Hochberg's, impose less stringent adjustments in order to increase power, but they still generally work best when the number of comparisons is small, for example, less than 20, and when the effect size is large (9,10). In fact, with a large number of comparisons, it is more efficient to accept a certain percentage of false positives and control the FDR, i.e., the fraction of false positive inferences. Methods that control FDR, e.g., Benjamini–Hochberg (BH) and Storey's corrections, are more sensitive than FWER methods, the latter of which sacrifice power to control false positives (9,10). The choice of correction method therefore depends on the number of comparisons, and the acceptable ratio of false positives with regard to the research question and study design. In general, when the significance threshold and null hypothesis are fixed, multiple testing by FDR correction yields more significant results in most cases or at least as many significant results as using FWER correction (9,10). When engaged in a research study that involves multiple comparisons, advice from a biostatistics expert can be highly valuable and reduce issues with manuscript review.

What if we have more than one independent variable for analysis? Options are available in common statistical packages to handle these cases. For example:

- Two-way ANOVA: This allows analysis of two independent categorical variables and one continuous dependent variable. Consider the mouse experiment mentioned earlier and assume that we have, in Figure 3.10, the exact same conditions but we give each rat either a placebo or a drug that affects the pathway. We are still interested in the creatinine level (continuous dependent variable) but we now have three different rats (categorical independent variable) and two different drugs (categorical independent variable) to account for. Two-way ANOVA by definition has multiple comparison testing and results have to be reported in that context using post-test calculations.

- Multivariable linear regression: This regression method assesses the association between a continuous dependent variable and multiple categorical or continuous independent variables at the same time. This model will be discussed in greater detail in Chapter 5.

So far we have been focusing on methods applicable to numerical dependent variables. In the next section, we will switch gear and look at tests that can be done with categorical dependent variables.

■ EXAMPLE: TUMOR CHARACTERISTICS ASSOCIATED WITH BREAST NODAL METASTASIS

Studies have suggested that certain tumor features may be associated with metastasis in breast cancer (11).

Hypothetical Study

A research group ran a study on 300 patients with breast cancer in their institution to examine the association of tumor features with regional nodal metastasis. The study was not matched. Table 3.4 shows the tumor characteristics based on a hypothetical data set (**see online materials; available at www.demosmedical.com/pathology-data-sets**).

What test can be done for the comparison? The researchers did chi-square goodness-of-fit test to produce the test results. The null hypothesis is that there is no association between the two categorical variables being assessed. What the test does is comparing observed to expected frequencies in each category under the assumption of no association to compute a x^2 statistic, which follows a chi-square distribution.

The greater proportions of nodal metastasis associated with poorly differentiated tumor, pT3 stage and lymphovascular invasion (LVI) suggest that tumor grade, pT stage, and LVI are likely predictors (Table 3.4). This observation is supported by the respective P values, confirming that the univariable associations of axillary nodal metastasis with tumor grade

($P < .001$), pT stage ($P = .001$) and LVI ($P = .02$) are statistically significant. It should be noted that the test and the P value alone would not tell us which category(ies) in a particular variable is/are driving the associations, and hence examination of the data itself (not just the P value) is important.

CAVEATS

Small or no counts in cells: The chi-square approximation may not be reliable with cells with small counts, which often happens with very fine categories. It was suggested that in 2×2 tables, if any expected counts are less than five, then some other test should be used (12). With contingency tables larger than 2×2, then in order to use chi-square test, no more than 20% of the expected counts are less than five and all individual expected counts are one or greater (13). Other options to consider in such settings would be doing exact tests, such as Fisher's exact test, or to combine the categories, if appropriate.

Matched versus unmatched data: Examples include studies that make multiple measures of the same variable on the same patient, for example, matching biopsy with subsequent resection or matching blood measures of the same test, usually before and after a treatment is administered. In such cases, matched testing or modeling (e.g., McNemar's test or conditional logistic regression) needs to be done.

Presence of confounders: The aforementioned analysis shows only univariable associations between the tumor features and regional nodal metastasis. It is unclear whether the association is subject to confounding by just looking at the chi-square test outputs. This issue can be addressed via study design and/or data analysis. For example,

- Restricting recruitment of subjects by characteristics may be an option to eliminate unequal distribution of confounding factors across groups of comparison. The disadvantage is that factors that are being restricted for cannot have their effects on the outcome fully evaluated. In addition, such a study design limits generalizability of results and can still be subject to residual confounding not accounted for by the restriction criteria. For example, in our hypothetical study on the relationship between blood microRNAs and lymph node metastasis of breast cancer, we can exclude women who had oral estrogen prior to diagnosis, history of another cancer, or chemotherapy treatment if data suggest these are confounders for the associations of interest and we want to control them at the phase of study design.

(text continues on page 70)

TABLE 3.4
Tumor Characteristics in Study Population ($N = 300$; Hypothetical Data)

TUMOR CHARACTERISTICS	TOTAL $N = 300$ n (col %)	PRESENCE OF AXILLARY NODAL METASTASIS $N = 149$ n (col %)	NO AXILLARY NODAL METASTASIS $N = 151$ n (col %)	P
Tumor grade				<.001
Well differentiated	64 (21)	21 (14)	43 (29)	
Moderately differentiated	182 (61)	85 (57)	97 (64)	
Poorly differentiated	54 (18)	43 (29)	11 (7)	
pT stage				.005
T1	64 (21)	26 (17)	38 (25)	
T2	156 (52)	71 (48)	85 (56)	
T3	80 (27)	52 (35)	28 (18)	

(continued)

TABLE 3.4
Tumor Characteristics in Study Population (*N* = 300; Hypothetical Data) (*continued*)

TUMOR CHARACTERISTICS	TOTAL *N* = 300 *n* (col %)	PRESENCE OF AXILLARY NODAL METASTASIS *N* = 149 *n* (col %)	NO AXILLARY NODAL METASTASIS *N* = 151 *n* (col %)	*P*
Presence of lymphovascular invasion				.02
Yes	39 (13)	26 (17)	13 (9)	
No	261 (87)	123 (83)	138 (91)	
Hormone receptor status				.91
ER+/PR+	131 (44)	68 (46)	63 (42)	

(continued)

TABLE 3.4
Tumor Characteristics in Study Population (*N* = 300; Hypothetical Data) (*continued*)

TUMOR CHARACTERISTICS	TOTAL *N* = 300 *n* (col %)	PRESENCE OF AXILLARY NODAL METASTASIS *N* = 149 *n* (col %)	NO AXILLARY NODAL METASTASIS *N* = 151 *n* (col %)	*P*
ER+/PR−	107 (36)	52 (35)	55 (36)	
ER−/PR+	25 (8)	12 (8)	13 (9)	
ER−/PR−	37 (12)	17 (11)	20 (13)	

- Matching: We can ensure the study groups are the same with respect to confounders by matching on those characteristics. The data collected will be correlated and matched analyses need to be performed for the categorical outcomes of interest. This approach is useful when the outcome of interest is of low prevalence, or when the confounders are multifaceted variables, like heredity factors. The disadvantage with this method is that we cannot evaluate for the factors being matched for in the study. For example, in Table 3.4, if all women in the study who have axillary lymph node metastasis are matched by age and estrogen exposure history, then neither age nor estrogen exposure history can be evaluated between the groups.

- Stratification: We can stratify analysis by categories in which the confounding variable does not vary or varies a little. Stratum-specific effect estimates (usually relative risks or odds ratios) are calculated and then compared with the effect estimate in the whole study. The limitations are that the method can be laborious if there is more than one confounder to control for, and that it requires categorization of continuous confounders and introduces potential residual confounding. For example, in Table 3.4, we could evaluate all categories by age stratification in groups of decades (age 40–49, age 50–59, age 60–69, age 70 or older) if we thought age was confounding our primary associations.

- Multivariable regression analysis: This analytic method allows us to assess the association between the predictor and outcome variables, and to control for multiple confounders at the same time. We will go over this model in greater detail in Chapter 5.

■ FURTHER ISSUES TO CONSIDER IN COMPARATIVE TESTING: POWER, EFFECT SIZE, AND SAMPLE SIZE

Recent medical research reviews found that a significant percentage of reported studies are underpowered (14,15). Increased number of false negatives and reduced power are common pitfalls in genomic studies, and in studies with relatively small sample size due to either fiscal constraints, low prevalence of the condition being studied, or a small effect size being investigated.

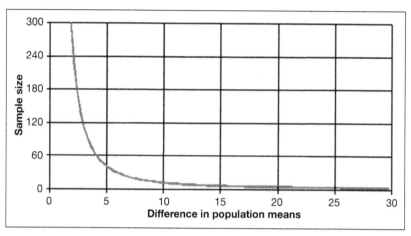

FIGURE 3.13
Relationship between sample size and effect size with difference in population means as an example (power set at 80% and α at 0.05).

Sample size and power calculation should be assessed in the phase of study design. Figure 3.13 shows the relationship between sample size and the effect size, taking an example of a two–independent-sample *t* test with power set at 80% and α at 0.05. We can see that as sample size increases, the effect size that the study can detect with sufficient power drops dramatically. Hence with a very large sample size, a statistically significant difference conveyed by a *P* value does not necessarily mean that the difference is clinically or biologically significant. The effect sizes and confidence intervals therefore should always be reported and considered along with the *P* value of a test (16). Sample size and power calculation will be discussed in further detail in Chapter 9.

■ LIMITATIONS OF COMPARATIVE STATISTICAL TESTS

Comparative tests can help us to reject a null hypothesis, but they cannot answer other questions in the study. For example: What are the odds that a hypothesis is correct? How strong is the association? Is the association confounded? Further statistical analysis and modeling, such as regression analysis, will need to be done to answer those questions. Regression analyses will be discussed further in Chapter 5.

TAKE-HOME POINTS

- The statistical methods used to make inferences on population parameters should be determined when we design the study and not after.
- A sample size that would give sufficient power to detect the hypothesized effect size should be identified before we set out to collect data.
- Every statistical test is associated with a null and an alternative hypothesis, which should be determined *before* conducting the tests.
- Know the definitions of *P* value, type I error (α), type II error (β), and power($1-\beta$).
- Type I error rate is prone to inflation in multiple hypothesis testing and α needs to be corrected before multiple testing is performed.
- Selection of a comparative test is based on study design, data type, and data distribution.
- Significance of a test output should not be interpreted solely based on the *P* values but should also be based on the effect size and estimated confidence intervals.

QUESTIONS FOR SELF-STUDY

1. Which of the following represents an example of ordinal data?

    A. Temperature measured in Celsius

    B. Gleason grade (grade 3, grade 4, and grade 5)

    C. Type of esophageal cancer (adenocarcinoma, squamous cell carcinoma, adenoid cystic carcinoma, etc.)

    D. Preferred alcoholic beverage (beer, wine, or liquor)

    E. Serum cholesterol

2. Parametric tests (*t* tests) and nonparametric tests (Wilcoxon rank-sum test) for a study:

    A. Should be utilized by whichever gives the best *P* value.

B. Must be decided upon and used, one or the other, for the whole study.

C. Should be dictated by the natural distribution of the data for each variable.

D. Can be decided upon after all data are collected and some preliminary analyses are done.

E. Are not important for determining variables in logistic regression models.

3. A study is designed where patients with a mesothelioma of either the pleural cavity or the peritoneal cavity have their tumors scored for number of mitoses per number of cells positive for keratin. Which of the following is an appropriate statistical measurement for the data?

A. t test of means

B. Wilcoxon rank-sum test

C. Poisson counting test

D. Logistic regression

E. Chi-square test

4. A new mouse model of cholangiocarcinoma is created using a gene knockout in the presence of a small molecule, and the reporter method is total fluoresence intensity (measured as a continuous variable) of the whole mouse at 10 weeks. If we wanted to show that the knockout with the small molecule is driving the tumor burden (as reflected by the total intensity fluorescence), what sort of statistical test/model should we use?

A. Logistic regression with fluoresence intensity as dependent variable.

B. Linear regression with knockout mouse as the dependent variable.

C. Two-way ANOVA with fluoresence intensity as the dependent variable.

D. Fisher's exact test for mouse versus small molecule.

E. Wilcoxon signed-rank test.

Questions 5 and 6 are based on the following hypothetical study:

A group of researchers did a clinical trial to study the effect of parenteral ascorbic acid in combination with conventional chemotherapy in patients with recurrent platinum-sensitive ovarian cancer. They designed two different dosing regimens (regimen 1 or regimen 2) of ascorbic acid for the trial and divided patients into three groups who received the following treatments: (a) conventional chemotherapy only, (b) conventional chemotherapy + ascorbic acid regimen 1, or (c) conventional chemotherapy + ascorbic acid regimen 2. Subgroup analyses were also done based on the chemotherapy regimens used. One of the parameters they measured in these patients was serum CA125 level at baseline and at follow-ups after treatment.

5. They compared the mean levels of serum CA125 in these patients after the first round of treatments by ANOVA. Which of the following is the hypothesis they tested by using this test?

   A. The mean level of CA125 is higher in those groups receiving ascorbic acid.

   B. The mean level of CA125 is the same across the groups after the first round of treatment.

   C. The mean level of CA125 is associated with ascorbic acid treatment.

   D. The mean level of CD125 is different in at least two of the groups after the first round of treatment.

   E. There is no hypothesis associated with this test.

6. A P value was yielded by the ANOVA test. Is it appropriate to use 0.05 as the significance threshold to interpret this P value?

   A. Yes. It is okay to use 0.05 as the significance threshold as it is what is conventionally used for all statistical tests.

   B. Yes. It is okay to use 0.05 as the significance threshold as it is what should always be used for ANOVA.

   C. No, using 0.05 as the significance threshold would lead to inflation of the type II error.

   D. No, using 0.05 as the significance threshold would lead to inflation of the type I error.

   E. Unable to determine as the significance threshold should be set based on the analytic results of the observed data.

Questions 7 and 8 are based on the following hypothetical study:

A cross-sectional study was done to evaluate the association between smoking and colorectal cancer. Patients who presented to a colonoscopy clinic in a tertiary hospital for colon biopsies in the past 15 years were included in this study. Primary outcome of interest was diagnosis of colorectal adenocarcinoma. Patients' smoking exposure was characterized as never/ever smokers. Information was also collected on pathologic tumor stage (pT: 0, Tis, 1, 2, 3, 4) at diagnosis among those who underwent resections. Patients who had recurrent colorectal cancer were excluded from the study.

7. Which of the following would be an appropriate test to examine the univariable association between smoking exposure and pT stage among those who did not receive neoadjuvant chemotherapy before their tumor resection?

   A. Pearson correlation coefficient

   B. Paired *t* test

   C. Chi-square test

   D. McNemar's test

   E. Log-rank test

8. The appropriate test was performed. A *P* value was obtained. Which of the following is true of this *P* value?

   A. If the $P < .5$, then smoking exposure and colorectal adenocarcinoma are causally associated.

   B. If the $P = .02$, then there is a 2% probability that the observed association is merely due to chance.

   C. If the $P = .05$, then there is a 5% probability that the null hypothesis is true.

   D. If the $P = .05$, then there is a 5% probability that the alternative hypothesis is wrong.

   E. If the $P = .05$, then, if the null hypothesis were true (i.e., no association between smoking exposure and pT stage of colorectal adenocarcinoma), we would see only 5% of repeated samples from the population having the same or greater observed association between smoking and colorectal cancer.

ANSWERS TO QUESTIONS FOR SELF-STUDY

1. Answer: B. Ordinal data are a type of categorical data in which the variable subcategories can be meaningfully ordered. In the examples, B, C, and D are all categorical variables; however, whereas Gleason grades can be meaningfully ordered in numerical fashion, there is no meaningful order to general types of esophageal cancer or preferred alcoholic beverage. Temperature and serum cholesterol represent continuous variables.

2. Answer: C. Normally distributed variables in a data set (Gaussian or near-Gaussian) should be tested with parametric tests. Nonnormal data or skewed data should be analyzed with nonparametric tests. These decisions are made *before* any analysis is done.

3. Answer: C. In this case, the number of mitoses is counted per the number of cells. If only raw mitoses per case were used, *t* test or rank sum might be correct. Logistic regression is appropriate for a yes/no outcome in relation to continuous or categorical dependent variables but not counting variables. Poisson counting must be used and will be discussed in a later chapter.

4. Answer: C. Logistic regression requires a categorical outcome variable and fluoresence intensity is continuous. Linear regression requires a continuous outcome variable and knockout mouse is categorical. A Fisher's exact test would not be appropriate because the outcome variable is a continuous variable. Wilcoxon signed-rank test is for paired nonparametric data and we do not have paired mice. A two-way ANOVA is correct because we have two mice (wild type and knockout) and for each mouse and we have two conditions for assessment (presence or absence of small molecule) in the two groups of mice. In this example, one experimental hypothesis could be that the fluorescence intensity (reflecting tumor burden) is significantly higher in knockout mice in the presence of small molecule than the other groups.

5. Answer: B. Choice B is the null hypothesis for the ANOVA test in this setting. Choice D is incorrect. The alternative hypothesis in this case should be that the mean level of CA125 is different in at least two, not three, of the patient groups. Choice E is incorrect

as there is a hypothesis associated with this statistical test. Choices A and C are incorrect as those are not what ANOVA is testing.

6. Answer: D. Type I error is the error made when a true null hypothesis is erroneously rejected. Pairwise comparisons are made with ANOVA with the three patient groups in this question. If we assume a reference statistical significance level of 0.05 for this ANOVA, the type I error rate will be inflated to 14% (i.e., $1-(1-0.05)^3$). Hence both choice A and choice B are incorrect. Choice C is incorrect as it is the type I, not type II, error that would be affected in this case. Choice E is incorrect as the significance threshold should be set a priori for statistical analyses.

7. Answer: C. The variables being evaluated (pT stage and smoking exposure) are both categorical variables. Hence choices A and B are incorrect as both tests pertain to continuous variables. Choice D is incorrect as the samples observed in this study are independent of each other. McNemar's test is relevant in case-control study settings or when data are matched on other characteristics. Choice E, log-rank test, is for comparing Kaplan–Meier survival functions and is not relevant in this cross-sectional study.

8. Answer: E. Choice A is incorrect as P value does not prove causality. Choices B, C, and D are incorrect as P value is not the probability that the null hypothesis is true, nor is it a probability that the observed association is due to chance. Choice D is incorrect as the P value does not tell us the probability that the alternative hypothesis is wrong. Choice E is correct as that is the definition of P value in this setting.

◼ REFERENCES

1. Krzywinski M, Altman N. Points of significance: comparing samples—part I. *Nat Methods*. 2014;11(3):215-216.
2. Krzywinski M, Altman N. Points of significance: nonparametric tests. *Nat Methods*. 2014;11(5):467-468.
3. Snell EJ. A scaling procedure for ordered categorical data. *Biometrics*. 1964;20(3):592-607.

4. van Rosmalen J, Koning AJ, Groenen PJ. Optimal scaling of interaction effects in generalized linear models. *Multivariate Behav Res.* 2009;44(1):59-81.

5. McGuire A1, Brown JA, Kerin MJ. Metastatic breast cancer: the potential of miRNA for diagnosis and treatment monitoring. *Cancer Metastasis Rev.* 2015;34(1):145-155.

6. Liu S, Guo W, Han X, et al. Role of UBIAD1 in intracellular cholesterol metabolism and vascular cell calcification. *PLOS ONE.* 2016;11(2):e0149639.

7. Cumming G, Fidler F, Vaux DL. Error bars in experimental biology. *J. Cell Biol.* 2007;177:7-11.

8. Sham PC, Purcell SM. Statistical power and significance testing in large-scale genetic studies. *Nat Rev Genet.* 2014;15(5):335-346.

9. Noble WS. How does multiple testing correction work? *Nat Biotechnol.* 2009;27(12):1135-1137.

10. Krzywinski M, Altman N. Points of significance: comparing samples—part II. *Nat Methods.* 2014;11(4):355-356.

11. Chen W, Cai F, Zhang B, et al. The level of circulating miRNA-10b and miRNA-373 in detecting lymph node metastasis of breast cancer: potential biomarkers. *Tumour Biol.* 2013;34(1):455-462.

12. Cochran WG. Some methods for strengthening the common chi square tests. *Biometrics.* 1954;10:417-451.

13. Moore DS, McCabe GP, Yates D. *The Practice of Statistics.* New York: W. H. Freeman & Company; 1999:734.

14. Button KS, Ioannidis JP, Mokrysz C, et al. Power failure: why small sample size undermines the reliability of neuroscience. *Nat Rev Neurosci.* 2013;14(5):365-376.

15. Breau RH, Carnat TA, Gaboury I. Inadequate statistical power of negative clinical trials in urological literature. *J Urol.* 2006;176(1):263-266.

16. Gelman A. Stern H. The difference between "significant" and "not significant" is not itself statistically significant. *Am Stat.* 2006;60:328-331.

CHAPTER 4

Concordance Analyses

Douglas A. Mata
Danny A. Milner Jr.

■ INTRODUCTION

Describing the relationship one variable has with another is a concept broadly referred to as "statistical dependence" or "correlation." This concept is very easy to appreciate in our everyday lives in the following examples: number of dollars spent on gasoline is inversely correlated with an automobile's fuel efficiency rating; the number of miles per hour over the speed limit you drive is positively correlated with the fine you will pay if caught; the rarity of a food item on a menu is correlated with the price you pay; and the amount of water and sunshine your garden receives is positively correlated with plant growth. Now let's imagine an example relevant to pathology. We have put together a data set of 56 cases of individuals diagnosed with retroperitoneal liposarcomas (provided as chapter 4-1.csv; **available at www.demosmedical .com/pathology-data-sets**). Each case has been input into a separate row in your spreadsheet, and each column contains data for a different variable. Let's import our data into R and take a peek at the first six rows of our spreadsheet (Figure 4.1).

We hypothesize that patient body mass index (BMI) is correlated with the mass of the resection specimen at final pathology. There are a number of ways that we could take these data columns—one for BMI and one for tumor mass—and compare and contrast them to see if any relationship or trend exists. For this example, there might be a biologically plausible relationship between patient size and tumor weight.

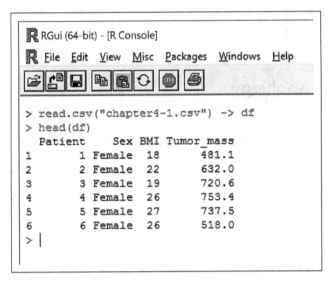

FIGURE 4.1
Fifty-six patients with data on sex, BMI, and retroperitoneal liposarcoma mass.

What should we do first? Although this chapter is about correlations, we shouldn't forget what we learned in Chapter 2. First we should look at our variables of interest. A simple way to compare the relationship between two variables is to plot them against one another. In R, we can type `plot(df$BMI, df$Tumor_mass)` to do this. In Stata, we can type **graph twoway scatter BMI Tumor_mass** (Figure 4.2).

In this particular example, we can clearly see that tumor mass increases with BMI. What if we wanted to summarize this relationship in a quantitative manner? We could calculate a correlation coefficient, that is, a measure of the strength and direction of a linear relationship between two variables. In R, we can calculate Pearson's correlation coefficient easily by simply typing `cor(df$BMI, df$Tumor_mass, method = "pearson")` and in Stata we just use the command **corr BMI Tumor_mass**. Or, we can calculate Spearman's correlation coefficient by modifying the code slightly, as shown in Figure 4.3, or in Stata using the command **spearman BMI Tumor_mass**. In either case, the resulting correlation ranges from −1 to +1 where 0 is no correlation, positive numbers are positive (or direct) correlation, and negative numbers are negative (or inverse) correlations. We revisit this method in more detail later.

Our result, 0.67, is what we would expect it to be given the shape of our graph. There is a moderately strong, positive relationship between

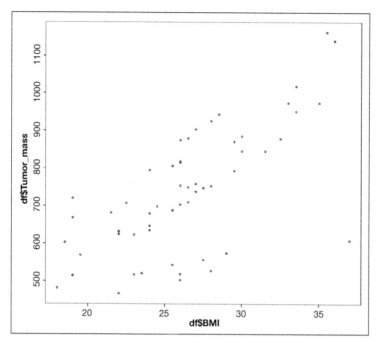

FIGURE 4.2
BMI versus tumor mass in patients with liposarcomas.

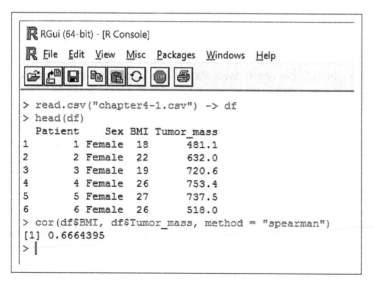

FIGURE 4.3
Calculating Spearman's correlation coefficient.

the variables. Based on this result, we might speculate that obesity *causes* increased tumor mass. However, we must keep in mind that merely measuring the correlation between these two variables is not in and of itself sufficient to establish cause and effect. We could instead more correctly conclude that overweight patients are more prone to being diagnosed with heavier tumors, without making any judgment as to causality.

In making this conclusion, we remember that "correlation is not causation." The classic example of this mistake is the fact that the number of cups of coffee people drink per day is correlated with lung cancer incidence. However, we would be remiss to assume that coffee drinking causes cancer. In fact, coffee intake per day also happens to be correlated with cigarette smoking, which in fact causes lung cancer. This is an example of "confounding," and we do not want to make this classic error when interpreting our own results using correlation and agreement analyses. Now, let's have a look at what these terms mean in a statistical context.

◼ DEFINING CORRELATION AND AGREEMENT

It is worth momentarily considering the basic definitions of correlation and agreement. Correlation is an attempt to assess a relationship, usually a linear one, between variables. The term "correlation" refers specifically to a relationship or connection between *two* different variables (not three or four variables), just like in our BMI and tumor mass example. It is often referred to as a quantity that measures the extent of "interdependence" between two variables. Agreement, a similar but different concept, refers to harmony or accordance in opinion or feeling, in other words, consistency. A practical example would be if you were to give a hundred lung cancer slides to two different pathologists and compare how often they agreed on the presence of lymphovascular invasion. As touched upon earlier, merely examining the correlation or agreement between two variables makes no judgment about causality. It makes no attempt to predict the behavior or outcome of one variable due to another. Of course, there may indeed be a causal connection at play—for example, in our example of patient BMI and tumor mass—and investigating that will be the subject of later chapters.

Pearson's Correlation Coefficient and Spearman's Rank Correlation

As we just learned, Pearson's correlation coefficient (also known as the interclass correlation coefficient, and abbreviated as "r") allows us to describe the linear relationship between two variables, and yields a value between +1 and −1. For our example of BMI and tumor mass, since tumor mass tended to increase with BMI, but did not do so perfectly, the correlation coefficient was positive but not quite 1. Some statisticians recommend that you use Pearson's correlation coefficient only on paired data that are two measures (continuous or categorical) of the same value. An example of this would be examining the correlation between Her2 immunohistochemical staining and evidence of Her2 amplification by fluorescence in situ hybridization (FISH).

How do we interpret Pearson's correlation coefficient? It's important to know that it is sensitive to outliers and to the distribution of data, and that guidelines for interpretation are arbitrary and also contextual. For example, an r of 0.85 may be considered low if using high-sensitivity measures but may be considered very high if using subjective, low-sensitivity measures. The nonparametric counterpart to Pearson's coefficient is Spearman's rank correlation, which assumes a monotonic relationship between variables. Implementing this test in R is simple. We can simply modify our earlier code by writing `cor (df$BMI, df$Tumor_mass, method = "spearman")` or using the Stata command **spearman BMI Tumor_mass**. Now that we have discussed correlation, let's tackle reproducibility (i.e., agreement).

Measuring Agreement With the Kappa Statistic

The kappa statistic provides a means of measuring the agreement between or among two or more reviewers. So if we had two different pathologists determine the grade of the same 100 slides of adenocarcinoma, we could calculate their kappa to see how well they agreed with one another. The kappa attempts to correct for agreement due merely to chance. There are several "types" of kappas, with names like Cohen's kappa, two-rater or multirater kappa, Light's kappa, Fleiss's kappa, and so forth, all slightly modified to deal with different situations and data types. The kappa statistic is used only for dealing with categorical data—not continuous data. When you calculate a kappa statistic between two categorical variables, you will get a number between zero and one. Interpretation of this output is somewhat arbitrary, but here are several guidelines:

κ statistic:

0 = no agreement

0–0.20 = slight agreement

0.20–0.40 = fair agreement

0.40–0.60 = moderate agreement

0.60–0.80 = substantial agreement

0.80–1.0 = near-perfect agreement

If your adenocarcinoma data set provided a kappa of 0.65, you might conclude that there is 0.65 agreement among reviewers on the evaluation of adenocarcinoma grade. Let's work through an example together using the vignette provided here.

Vignette for Understanding the Kappa Statistic

While investigating enzymes responsible for branched-chain fatty acid metabolism in liver cells, you identify a novel protein that appears to interact with alpha-methylacyl-CoA racemase (AMACR), an enzyme involved in fatty acid metabolism. Reading about AMACR, you discover that it is used diagnostically in prostate cancer pathology, as it is overexpressed in the majority of prostate cancers but not in benign prostate tissue. Realizing that your novel protein may also be overexpressed in prostate cancer, you hypothesize that expression of your novel protein may also have diagnostic utility in prostate cancer.

Working with the urologist at your institution, you obtain 20 transurethral resection of the prostate (TURP) specimens that were obtained after surgical intervention to relieve obstructive symptoms. The specimens all contain benign prostate tissue. Likewise, you obtain 20 treatment-refractory prostate cancer metastasis samples. After validating the performance of an antibody against your novel protein using positive and negative control cell lines, you perform immunohistochemistry for expression of your novel protein on the 40 samples. You find moderate to strong staining in the majority of cancer cells in 18 of 20 prostate cancer metastasis samples, and weak staining in benign prostate epithelial cells in only one of 20 TURP specimens. Based on these results, you conclude that expression of your novel protein may have utility in diagnosing prostate cancer.

One of the major areas to consider when evaluating the potential utility of a diagnostic biomarker is the area of intended clinical use. This often requires a deep understanding of the clinical issues regarding the diagnosis of the disease you are interested in, and will likely require consultation or collaboration with clinical experts. One of the most critical aspects to consider when planning the evaluation of a novel diagnostic biomarker is the current diagnostic process for the disease. For example, the majority of men in the United States diagnosed with prostate cancer were identified from the population by an elevated level of serum prostate specific antigen (PSA), which prompted a transrectal ultrasound-guided biopsy of the prostate, where multiple small cores of prostatic tissue are obtained with histopathologic evaluation by a pathologist. Most series find that about 30% to 40% of men undergoing prostate biopsy in the United States are found to have prostate cancer on biopsy. In diagnostically challenging cases, the pathologist most commonly will utilize immunohistochemistry for basal cell markers (which are lost in prostate cancer) and AMACR (which is overexpressed in most prostate cancers).

Prior to submitting your findings for publication and releasing a statement claiming that you have discovered a novel diagnostic biomarker for prostate cancer that you expect will be used in practice soon, you need to evaluate whether assessment of your diagnostic biomarker is reproducible. The most common method to evaluate the reproducibility of a diagnostic biomarker is by assessing interobserver agreement as assessed by the kappa statistic. Assessing interobserver agreement is particularly relevant for your biomarker, as subjective staining differences are described (weak versus moderate to strong), which may be interpreted differently by individuals.

A kappa of 1 indicates perfect agreement, whereas a kappa of 0 indicates agreement equivalent to chance. To determine the kappa statistic for your cohort of 100 prostate biopsy specimens with cancer, you could record the staining intensity in each specimen (negative, weak, moderate, strong) by two different pathologists. To simplify this example, we consider negative and weak to be "negative," and moderate and strong to be "positive."

The two pathologists agree that 87 of the cores are positive and four are negative. So their simple "percent agreement" is 91%. The percent agreement is defined as the percentage of events where two observers agree on a measurement. It's not used much due to its limitations; in particular, it does not account for agreement attributable simply to chance, and will be high if events that represent disagreement are rare. To calculate the more informative kappa statistic, construct a 2 × 2 table:

Observer 2	Observer 1		
	Biomarker +	Biomarker −	Total
Biomarker +	A	B	r
Biomarker −	C	D	s
Total	t	u	A+B+C+D=n

Observer 2	Observer 1		
	Biomarker +	Biomarker −	Total
Biomarker +	87	3	90
Biomarker −	6	4	10
Total	93	7	100

How do we calculate kappa? As mentioned earlier, the kappa statistic measures the difference between how much agreement is actually present ("observed" agreement) and how much agreement would be expected by chance ("expected" agreement).

The observed agreement is $(A + D)/n = 0.91$.

The expected agreement is more complicated to calculate:

Expected agreement $= [(t/n) \times (r/n)] + [(u/n) \times (s/n)]$

Expected agreement $= [(93/100) \times (90/100)] + [(7/100) \times (10/100)]$

Expected agreement $= 0.84$

Kappa $=$ (observed − expected)$/(1 -$ expected$) = 0.44$

So our result of 0.44 actually indicates that we just have moderate agreement. Now, you don't have to resort to pencil-and-paper mathematics to calculate kappa values for your research. Instead, we can do it in R or in Stata. Locate the file available at **www.demosmedical .com/pathology-data-sets**, entitled "chapter4-2.txt" and import it into the R workspace. Let's glance at the last six rows, and then tabulate their diagnoses (Figure 4.4).

As you can see, we have the results of the observations made by our two pathologists. They agree in 91 (i.e., 87 + 4) and disagree in 9 (i.e., 5 + 4) cases, similar to our prior example. We can use the fsmb package in R to estimate Cohen's kappa, and to test the null hypothesis that the extent of agreement is the same as random. First, let's install and load the package.

```
install.packages("fmsb")
library(fmsb)
```

The function in the package that we use is called Kappa.test(). You have to capitalize the "K" for it to work! Let's perform the kappa test on our two columns of data.

```
> Kappa.test(df$Pathologist_1, df$Pathologist_2)
$Result
Estimate Cohen's kappa statistics and test the null
hypothesis that the extent of agreement is same as
random (kappa = 0)
```

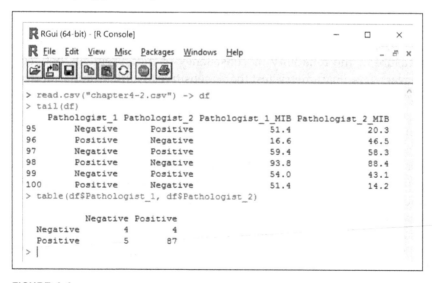

FIGURE 4.4
Diagnoses and MIB indexes rendered by two different pathologists.

```
data: df$Pathologist_1 and df$Pathologist_2
Z = 1.8098, P-value = 0.03517
95 percent confidence interval:
  0.06111443 0.78207323
sample estimates:
[1] 0.4215938
```

Here we can see that our kappa is 0.42, quite similar to the value of 0.44 that we got by hand in our prior example (the numbers differ slightly due to the weighting assumptions that R makes). To perform the same test in Stata, use the **kappa** command. What's nice about R's output is that it not only gives us the kappa of 0.42, but also gives us the upper and lower confidence intervals for kappa, 0.06 to 0.78. This wide range drives home the point that with only two pathologists and only 100 cases, the precision to which we can determine kappa in this case really isn't that great. We can also conclude that the extent of agreement between our two pathologists isn't just due to chance, given that we have a significant P value of .035.

The Intraclass Correlation Coefficient

We just learned how to measure agreement in measurements of binary categorical data made by two different observers. Now let's learn how to measure the consistency between measurements of continuous data made by different observers using the intraclass correlation coefficient (ICC). The ICC is a statistic that is useful for continuous data and is a measure of the reliability or consistency of measurements between observers. It is a parametric test that is sensitive to outliers and is perfect for continuous data. The ICC also gives an output between zero and one, just like the kappa statistic, with zero implying no consistency and one implying absolute consistency.

An important limitation is that exchangeability must hold between observers; otherwise our results may be obscured by intraobserver variations. Exchangeability is a somewhat difficult concept to apply to pathologists—it doesn't necessarily mean that one pathologist can be exchanged for another, but it does imply that there is less potential for substantially different evaluation, meaning that "exchangeable" pathologists are likely to have a similar number of years of experience, are likely to have possibly trained or continue to practice in a similar or the same environment, and are likely to have a similar level of subspecialty training (if applicable). Another way to think about this is that if we were comparing a first-year anatomic pathology resident to a senior pathologist with 20 years of experience, we could refer to the senior pathologist as the "gold standard" and, thus, these two observers are not interchangeable. Whether exchangeability holds is a subjective decision, and the parameters used to make this decision may vary in importance for different diagnoses. For example, if there is significant regional variation in assessment of a particular feature on a particular kind of biopsy, including two pathologists from different regions in a study might call into question whether exchangeability holds for this situation. Remember, the concept of exchangeability must hold in order for measures of agreement to be truly valid. If reviewers are not "exchangeable," then the measure will be obscured by interobserver variations.

Let's return to our previous data set. In the same spreadsheet, we have two other columns, each containing the Ki-67/MIB-1 proliferation index (a percentage between 0% and 100%) estimated by the two pathologists. The variables are named `Pathologist_1_MIB` and `Pathologist_2_MIB`, respectively. To calculate the ICC, we need to install and load the `ICC` package, and then use the `ICCest()` function. Calculating the ICC is just as simple in R as was calculating kappa, as shown in the following.

```
> ICCest(df$Pathologist_1_MIB, df$Pathologist_2_MIB)
$ICC
[1] 0.9212543
$LowerCI
[1] 0.6195287
$UpperCI
[1] 0.9689997
$N
[1] 94
$k
[1] 1.063226
$varw
[1] 73.39667
$vara
[1] 858.6753

Warning message:
In ICCest(df$Pathologist_1_MIB, df$Pathologist_2_MIB) :
  'x' has been coerced to a factor
```

Don't worry about the warning message at the bottom. The dependent variable in this test must be coded as a factor for R to interpret it, and it has done this automatically for you. The command in Stata is **icc**. Let's have a look at our results. We can state that there is 0.92 consistency among observers in evaluation of the MIB-1 index. As before, we get a confidence interval (0.62–0.97) for our statistic, emphasizing the degree to which our result is (or isn't) precise.

■ PRACTICAL CONSIDERATIONS BEFORE BEGINNING YOUR STUDY

When a study is designed to compare how well one person does against another (competition), we use statistics that have a "gold standard" and compare all others to that. When we are interested in agreement (because we want to create criteria that anyone can use) there are a few tools that are available to us that are extremely important in ensuring validity to our system and, most importantly, reproducibility outside of our study design. The value of these tools is that they allow us to define criteria and standardize applications and are very likely to increase agreement, especially if there is substantial difference in reviewers. However, they are not needed for all studies.

Preview: In this design, a set of observers may look at the same set of cases (possibly together) to understand the range of a given variable and how the data are to be reported. They are not necessarily told that certain cases meet certain criteria. They are allowed to review cases so they have a sense of the parameters they are measuring. For example, a group of four residents are given 20 cases by a senior pathologist and told that the cases represent squamous intraepithelial neoplasia of the vulva and benign lesions. The group of four study the slides and understand the spectrum of case pathology before scoring actual cases.

Education: In this design, a group of future observers are taught by an expert observer about the system they are going to score, the different criteria, and, often, pitfalls in reviewing cases. An example may be residents attending a national conference led by a content expert where a new scoring system for a tumor is presented, and then volunteer attendees can score cases afterward to test agreement of the system.

Consensus meeting: In a consensus meeting, a group of observers (often a large group) discuss current criteria, guidelines, and rules for observing a given feature and determine hard criteria that are to be used for classification. These are quite common in pathology and, after such a meeting, having two or more observers attempt to apply these criteria to unknown cases is an excellent example of the statistics described earlier.

Study set(s): Similar to education, this is self-study of a set of prelabeled cases that, by some other means (e.g., gold standard, consensus, senior expert), have been classified. For example, if a department of pathology has a large set of 300 cases of all gynecologic lesions of the ovary in which three pathology residents review these cases independently, that would be an appropriate prestudy approach to then compare their agreement using the aforementioned statistics.

Adjudicated postreview: In this design, after all observers have scored their cases, discrepant cases are reviewed together and a final corrected value for a given variable is determined. This is an important finishing phase of a criteria design but would need to be revalidated should new rules arise. For example, if the same four residents now each score 200 cases of vulvar lesions, the 25 lesions on which any one of the group disagreed are reviewed together and a final group assessment is made about these cases. This could be done by the four residents or by two unrelated senior-level experts with the latter providing "gold standards" on which to compare the cases. Another important aspect of postreview is the ability to do additional tests not allowed during the observation phase to confirm problem diagnoses. These tools may then, in themselves, become part of the criteria used.

■ SUMMARY AND CONCLUSIONS

Now we have discussed percent agreement, kappa, and ICC, all of which give us ways to measure reproducibility in our data. Before that, we learned ways for measuring correlation, with sections on Pearson's correlation coefficient and Spearman's rank correlation. These techniques will serve you well as you analyze your data. In the next chapter, we discuss regression analysis.

TAKE-HOME POINTS

- Correlation is an attempt to assess a relationship, usually a linear one, between two variables.

- Agreement refers to reproducibility/consistency in measurements made by different observers.

- The kappa statistic is useful for measuring agreement in measurements of binary categorical data made by two different observers.

- The ICC is useful for measuring the consistency between measurements of continuous data made by different observers.

QUESTION FOR SELF-STUDY

1. Open the first data file that we used in this chapter, on the 56 patients with retroperitoneal liposarcomas. See if you can remember how to calculate Pearson's product-moment correlation coefficient between the variables BMI and tumor mass. What value do you get? Now, use R's built-in `help()` function to see if you can figure out how to calculate the 95% confidence interval for the correlation coefficient. Hint: have a look at the help file for the correlation coefficient function; it will point you in the right direction!

ANSWER TO QUESTION FOR SELF-STUDY

1. Calculating the product-moment correlation coefficient is simple; just type `cor(df$BMI, df$Tumor_mass, method = "pearson")` into the R prompt. To get help on the `cor()` command, type `help(cor)`. Under the "See also" section, the page will point you to another related command, `cor.test()`. You can apply the function in the same way; simply type `cor.test(df$BMI, df$Tumor_mass)` into the command prompt. This will provide you with the 95% confidence interval for the coefficient as well as test the hypothesis that the true correlation is not equal to zero.

■ RECOMMENDED READING

R Core Team. R: A language and environment for statistical computing. R Foundation for Statistical Computing, Vienna, Austria; 2015. Available at https://www.R-project.org

StataCorp. *Stata Statistical Software: Release 14*. College Station, TX: StataCorp LP; 2015. Available at: http://www.cookbook-r.com/Statistical_analysis/Inter-rater_reliability

CHAPTER 5

Regression Analyses in Cross-Sectional Studies: Logistic and Linear Regression

T. Rinda Soong
Danny A. Milner Jr.

■ INTRODUCTION

In Chapter 3, we discussed statistical hypothesis testing for sample comparison, which allows us to make crude inferences on whether there is an association between two variables or a difference of effects in populations. In this chapter, we examine how regression helps us further define the relationship between parameters of interest in the population. Rather than attempting to address every technical detail related to regression, which is a vast topic meriting at least a whole separate book, this chapter aims to highlight the principles and basic practical considerations in the context of logistic regression and general linear regression, which are the two most common regression models encountered in medical cross-sectional studies. In this chapter, we will first outline the basic steps involved in regression modeling, and then discuss these concepts in greater detail with the use of examples. References are provided at the end of this chapter for advanced reading.

■ WHAT IS A REGRESSION MODEL?

Regression analysis models the relationship between the outcome of interest and the predictor(s), thereby provides a reasonable approximation of the observed data pattern, and yields estimates for the population parameters of interest. Consider assessing the relationship between age and presentation of osteosarcoma. Previously in Chapter 3, we learned that we can compare age (continuous dependent variable) between those with and without osteosarcoma (categorical independent variable) in a univariable analysis using a *t* test of means. But what if we also want to see if gender, history of radiation, bone location, and history of trauma relates to the presence of osteosarcoma? In fact, we may be more interested in the presence or absence of osteosarcoma given any/all of these variables. Regression allows us to select a dependent variable (presence or absence of osteosarcoma) and then look at the effects of all independent variables at the same time. If we assess osteosarcoma as the dependent variable (a categorical variable), a logistic regression can be applied. If we want instead to evaluate the association between clinical features with the age of diagnosis of osteosarcoma (a continuous variable), a linear regression model would be more appropriate.

Regression models can be parametric, semiparametric, and nonparametric. Nonparametric regression is an analysis in which the predictor data distribution is constructed based on the observed data and not predetermined. For example, nonparametric regression includes nonparametric multiplicative regression (NPMR), which is often used in environmental studies, and classification and regression trees (CARTs), which will be discussed further in Chapter 8 (1). Semiparametric regression models have both parametric and nonparametric components, relaxing assumptions in full parametric models (2,3).

In this chapter, we focus on parametric regression analyses, which constitute the most frequently used methods by far in medical cross-sectional studies. Numerous types of models have been developed for different data types as well as different data distributions. Table 5.1 gives a summary of the characteristics of the most common regression models reported in literature for continuous, categorical, and count outcome data.

It should be noted that all the models listed in Table 5.1 are generalized linear models (GLMs)—a term which should not be confused with the general linear regression model. A GLM generalizes linear regression by allowing the model to be related to the response variable via a link function, and thereby unifying the model with different regressions, such as general linear regression, logistic regression, and so on. GLM is based on an iteratively reweighted least squares method for maximum likelihood estimation of the model parameters (4).

TABLE 5.1
Characteristics of Common Regression Models

MODEL	DATA TYPE OF DEPENDENT VARIABLE (Y)	DATA TYPE(S) OF INDEPENDENT VARIABLES (X)	EFFECT MEASURE	ASSUMPTIONS
General linear regression: $Y = \beta_0 + \beta_1 X_1 + \beta_2 X_2 \ldots + \varepsilon$	Continuous data	Numerical/ continuous/ categorical	Unit change of dependent variable	• Linear relationship between the outcome (Y) and predictor (X): • Y is a measured (continuous) variable = $\beta_0 + \beta_1 X_1 + \beta_2 X_2 \ldots + \beta_n X_n$ • Y has a normal distribution measured at any particular mean (μ) • Y has equal variance (σ^2) at any particular mean (μ) • Observations are independent of each other • These assumptions imply that the model errors are uncorrelated and normally distributed with mean 0 and variance σ^2
Logistic regression: $\text{logit}(p) = \beta_0 + \beta_1 X_1 \ldots + \varepsilon$	Categorical data	Categorical/ numerical/ continuous	Odds ratio	• The dependent variable of interest is a binary variable • Observations are independent of each other
Poisson regression: $\log_e(Y) = \beta_0 + \beta_1 X_1 \ldots + \varepsilon$	Count data	Categorical numerical/ continuous	Incident rate ratio	• The dependent variable of interest follows a Poisson distribution • Changes in the rate from combined effects of different predictors are multiplicative • At each level of the covariates, the number of cases has variance equal to the mean • Observations are independent of each other

General Steps in Regression Analysis

Regression modeling allows us to quantify the strength of an association and to include multiple predictors in one model to control for confounding and interaction. In general, there are three steps involved in regression analysis:

- Select a model appropriate for the data type and data distribution, and verify whether model assumptions are met
- Run and fit the model with predictor selection
- Run regression diagnostics and assess how well the model predicts the data

Model fitting involves running the model with a single predictor (univariable analyses) and multiple predictors (multivariable analyses). Note that there is a technical distinction between the terms *multivariable* regression and *multivariate* regression in statistical analyses even though these terms are often used interchangeably in literature (5): (a) A multivariable regression model refers to a model with two or more independent/predictor variables. (b) A multivariate regression model, in contrast, assesses the relationships between multiple dependent variables and a single set of predictor variables. This often happens with longitudinal studies or nested data.

Let us see how regression modeling works with some examples.

■ EXAMPLE: LOGISTIC REGRESSION

Hypothetical study

Interval colon cancers (colon cancers that were detected prior to the next recommended colonoscopy) are proposed to arise due to missed cancers in colonoscopy or a unique biologic pathway (6). A study group wanted to determine tumor characteristics associated with interval colon cancer. Data were from patients who underwent resections for colon adenocarcinoma. No matching was done. Table 5.2 shows the tumor features in relation to the interval status of colon cancer (hypothetical data set) (**see online materials; available at www.demosmedical.com/pathology-data-sets**). Based on the values there, interval colon cancer seems to be associated with the location of right colon and this P value was obtained by a chi-square test. Note, however, that although there seems to be a statistically significant association between tumor location and interval colon cancer ($P < .05$), we do not have a reportable effect size yet. The other features do not appear to be significant predictors (Table 5.2). Logistic regression is a reasonable

TABLE 5.2
Tumor Characteristics Associated With Interval Colon Cancer (N = 604; Hypothetical Data)

TUMOR CHARACTERISTICS	TOTAL N = 604 n (col %)	INTERVAL COLON CANCER N = 40 n (col %)	NON-INTERVAL COLON CANCER N = 564 n (col %)	P*
Tumor location				.004
Left colon (distal to splenic flexure)	372 (62)	16 (40)	356 (63)	
Right colon (proximal to splenic flexure)	232 (38)	24 (60)	208 (37)	
pT stage				.64
T1	59 (10)	6 (15)	53 (9)	
T2	135 (22)	8 (20)	127 (23)	
T3	279 (46)	19 (48)	260 (46)	
T4	131 (22)	7 (18)	124 (22)	
Regional nodal metastasis				.572
No	328 (54)	20 (50)	308 (54)	
Yes	276 (46)	20 (50)	256 (45)	
Presence of adenoma in resection				.84
No	282 (47)	18 (45)	264 (47)	
Yes	322 (53)	22 (55)	300 (53)	

*P values were obtained from chi-square goodness-of-fit test.

choice of model in this case to quantify the strength of the association (via producing a reportable effect size) between tumor location and interval status. It reports the difference in log odds (i.e., the odds ratio [OR]) associated with the predictor variable.

How can we determine the strength of the association? Figure 5.1A shows the univariable logistic regression output on tumor location and interval status of cancer using Stata with the command **logistic Interval Location (see online material available at www.demosmedical.com/ pathology-data-sets)**. In the data set, the left colon tumor is coded as "0" and is automatically treated as the reference category. The output tells us that a right colon tumor is associated with a 2.6-fold increase in odds of being interval cancer (95% CI: 1.3–4.9) as compared with a left colon tumor.

CAVEAT

Odds ratio versus relative risk: ORs should not be interpreted as if they were relative risks (RRs). The difference between OR and RR is illustrated in Figure 5.2. OR can be an approximation of RR when the prevalence

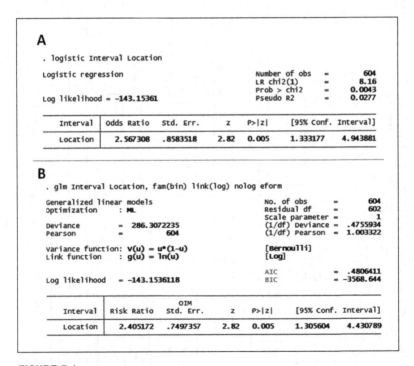

FIGURE 5.1

Univariable association of tumor location with interval cancer status, assessed by (A) logistic regression model and (B) generalized linear model.

	Outcome of interest		
Number		**+**	**−**
Exposure **+**		a	b
of interest **−**		c	d

$$RR = \frac{a/(a+b)}{c/(c+d)} \qquad OR = \frac{ad}{bc}$$

FIGURE 5.2
Distinction between odds ratio (OR) and relative risk (RR).

of outcome is low. It is important to keep in mind that when the prevalence of the outcome is high (> 10%), OR can become a significant overestimation of RR. In this particular example, the prevalence of the outcome (interval cancer) is small (6%) and the OR yielded by the logistic regression model is a good approximation of the RR, as confirmed by the output of a GLM model on tumor location and interval status (Figure 5.1B) given by the command **glm Interval Location, fam(bin) link(log) nolog eform**. Note that the **glm** command can give the estimate of RR but we need to specify that the distribution of the dependent variable interval is binomial (**fam(bin)**); that we want to use logistic regression (**link(log)**); we do not want to see the likelihood iterations (nolog) and we want estimates of RR (**eform**). When in Stata, typing "help glm" in the command line will produce a page describing all of the options for **glm**. Consider, however, the example in Chapter 3, which investigates the univariable association between axillary nodal metastasis and tumor grade: The prevalence of the outcome (nodal metastasis) is 50% in that example. If we compare the ORs and the RRs of the association between nodal metastasis and the different categories of tumor grade in that study, we would see that the point estimate of OR (OR: 8.0) associated with "_ITumor_gr~2" (poor differentiation relative to well differentiation) is markedly greater than that of the RR (RR: 2.4) (Figure 5.3). In such cases, ORs should never be taken as surrogates of RRs, and it may be more desirable to estimate the RRs directly using a model other than the logistic regression model (7–9). Note that running the model without the **xi** prefix and the **i.** prefix for **Tumor_grade** would produce a single OR estimate but the inclusion of this coding allows for interaction terms and factor expansion to look at point estimates at each level of the independent categorical variable.

A

```
. xi: logistic Metastasis i.Tumor_grade
i.Tumor_grade    _ITumor_gra_0-2    (naturally coded; _ITumor_gra_0 omitted)

Logistic regression                          Number of obs   =      300
                                             LR chi2(2)      =    28.76
                                             Prob > chi2     =   0.0000
Log likelihood = -193.55552                  Pseudo R2       =   0.0692
```

Metastasis	Odds Ratio	Std. Err.	z	P>|z|	[95% Conf. Interval]	
_ITumor_gr~1	1.794305	.5470391	1.92	0.055	.9871569	3.261419
_ITumor_gr~2	8.004329	3.443149	4.84	0.000	3.444858	18.59852

B

```
. xi: glm Metastasis i.Tumor_grade, fam(bin) link(log) nolog eform
i.Tumor_grade    _ITumor_gra_0-2    (naturally coded; _ITumor_gra_0 omitted)

Generalized linear models                    No. of obs       =       300
Optimization     : ML                        Residual df      =       297
                                             Scale parameter  =         1
Deviance         =  387.1110441              (1/df) Deviance  =  1.303404
Pearson          =  300.0000486              (1/df) Pearson   =  1.010101

Variance function: V(u) = u*(1-u)            [Bernoulli]
Link function    : g(u) = ln(u)              [Log]

                                             AIC              =   1.31037
Log likelihood   =  -193.555522              BIC              = -1306.912
```

Metastasis	Risk Ratio	OIM Std. Err.	z	P>|z|	[95% Conf. Interval]	
_ITumor_gr~1	1.423339	.2784228	1.80	0.071	.9700689	2.088401
_ITumor_gr~2	2.426809	.465108	4.63	0.000	1.66686	3.53323

FIGURE 5.3
Univariable association of nodal metastasis with tumor grade, assessed by (A) logistic regression model and (B) generalized linear model.

How to fit the model? We should first check for presence of collinearity among the variables. Inclusion of collinear variables generally does not affect the predictive power of the model as a whole for the outcome, but it may not give valid estimates about the predictive power of individual predictors. For example, assume we have a variable of hemoglobin and a variable of hematocrit in the same data set. These variables are expected to be very strongly (if not perfectly directly) correlated and, thus, would be collinear if we used them in the same model. There are several ways to check for collinearity, e.g. simple correlation matrices, looking at the standard error in a model output with and without the variables, and formal testing. Collinearity can be formally tested by looking at the variance inflation factor (VIF) with the use of statistical packages. Variables with high VIF (e.g., VIF > 10) need further investigation. There are no high values seen in this case and hence no suggestion of collinearity (Figure 5.4).

```
. vif
      Variable |      VIF        1/VIF
    ----------+---------------------------
             T |     1.19     0.838017
             N |     1.18     0.849096
      Location |     1.03     0.971004
       Adenoma |     1.02     0.984922
    ----------+---------------------------
      Mean VIF |     1.10
```

FIGURE 5.4

Check for collinearity among the variables of pT stage, pN stage, tumor location, and presence of adenoma in the data set.

After examining the outputs of univariable models between the outcome of interest and each predictor, we need to decide which of them should be included in the final model. The following are some issues that should be considered:

- **Is there confounding caused by any of the predictors on the primary association of interest?**
  One way to check it is to compare the effect estimates (the ORs or difference in log odds in logistic regression) associated with the primary predictor of interest before and after adding another predictor to the model. Confounding is present if the addition results in a significant change. In general, ≥10% is considered big enough but there is no hard-and-fast rule on that. One potential pitfall here is to mistake a mediator as a confounder and keep it in the model. Since the mediator is in the causal pathway underlying the association of interest (Figure 5.5), inclusion of such a variable in the model would lead to underestimation of the association effect. This can be avoided by having a good understanding of the research question and the related literature.

- **Is there evidence of interaction?**
  Suppose we suspect (not in this case based on exploratory and univariable analyses) the presence of adenoma may be an effect modifier of the association between tumor location and interval status of colon cancer. We can run a model to test if the OR associated with the interaction term "**Loc_Adenoma**" between the two is statistically significant (Figure 5.6). The interaction term (**Loc_Adenoma**) can be created using the command **gen**

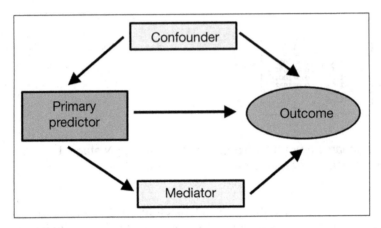

FIGURE 5.5
Schematic diagram showing the causal pathway and the relationship of confounder, mediator, the primary predictor and the outcome.

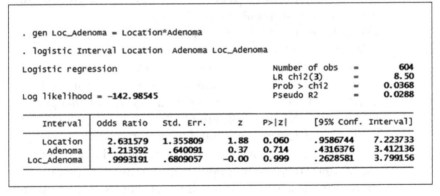

FIGURE 5.6
Check for interaction between tumor location and presence of adenoma.

Loc_Adenoma = Location*Adenoma. The **generate** (or in short form, **gen**) command is very valuable in Stata as it allows us to create variables de novo or from existing variables for a variety of reasons. As suggested by the model output, the OR associated with the term is not statistically significant and presence of interaction is not likely between these two variables (Figure 5.6). This process can be repeated for each variable to make sure no interaction is missed. Interaction testing can become quite cumbersome with larger models; however, this is a commonly omitted step in many research studies that should always be undertaken.

- **Are there any statistical tools that help with predictor selection to get a parsimonious model?**
  We can do likelihood ratio tests by comparing restricted and unrestricted models with a different number of predictors. Likelihood ratio test checks whether there is sufficient evidence to reject the null hypothesis that all of the regression coefficients for the added variables are zero. Statistical packages have built-in codes to run the process systematically by either adding more predictors into the model (forward selection) or removing predictors from the model (backward selection). Figure 5.7 shows the output of a backward selection starting with a model with all the variables—tumor location, T stage (**T**), presence of nodal metastasis (**N**), and presence of adenoma (**Adenoma**)—given by the command **sw logistic Interval Location Adenoma T N, pr(0.05) lr**. The components are **sw** (stepwise); **pr(0.05)**, which is the *P* value for each round of modeling that is used to remove variables; and **lr**, which performs the likelihood ratio test (as opposed to the Wald test, which is the default). All the variables fail the likelihood ratio test except tumor location in this example as it is the only variable remaining in the model after stepwise testing (Figure 5.7).

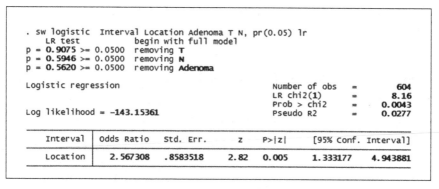

```
. sw logistic  Interval Location Adenoma T N, pr(0.05) lr
     LR test           begin with full model
 p = 0.9075 >= 0.0500  removing T
 p = 0.5946 >= 0.0500  removing N
 p = 0.5620 >= 0.0500  removing Adenoma

Logistic regression                        Number of obs   =       604
                                           LR chi2(1)      =      8.16
                                           Prob > chi2     =    0.0043
Log likelihood = -143.15361                Pseudo R2       =    0.0277
```

Interval	Odds Ratio	Std. Err.	z	P>|z|	[95% Conf. Interval]	
Location	2.567308	.8583518	2.82	0.005	1.333177	4.943881

FIGURE 5.7
Backward selection of predictors in a logistic regression model.

- **Is there literature evidence justifying any variable in the model?**
  This is perhaps the most important consideration in predictor selection as the model should be fitted and interpreted in the context of literature evidence and research background. The bottom line is that we should try to avoid simply dropping variable(s) from the model solely on the basis of the individual P values associated with the regression coefficients, or the difference of log odds in this example.

The Last Step: Model Checking and Regression Diagnostics

We can do a test to see how well the model is calibrated. Examples of such tests for logistic regression include Hosmer–Lemeshow test, which is most useful when there are many unique covariate patterns (combination of values of predictor variables) in the data. Pearson's goodness-of-fit test is another option, which is more useful when there are many nonunique covariate patterns in the data. The receiver operating characteristic (ROC) curve (plot of sensitivity vs. 1 – specificity) is a way to assess the discrimination of a fitted logistic model by looking at the classification statistics for specific cutoffs of predicted probabilities given by the model. It is useful for comparing competing classification schemes (based on different cutoffs) (10), and we can compare models by the ROC curves. The model with the highest area under the curve is the best at classification. Cross-validation and learning set/test set validation can be employed to avoid using the same individuals who fit the model to evaluate the performance of the classification schemes.

Other Types of Logistic Regression Models

Different logistic regression models have been developed to fit different data types and study designs. For example:

- Conditional logistic regression: useful for matched data

- Ordinal logistic regression: useful for ordinal dependent variables, e.g., quartiles of T-cell density in tumor

- Multinomial (aka polytomous) logistic regression: useful for categorical dependent variable with more than two unordered categories

▪ EXAMPLE: GENERAL LINEAR REGRESSION

Hypothetical Study

MicroRNAs (miRNAs) in blood have been suggested to be prognostic factors for metastatic breast cancer (11). A research group showed in a prior study that the ratio of miR-101/miR-25 (miR ratio) in blood of patients prior to lumpectomy is associated with axillary nodal metastasis. In this follow-up study, the researchers examined if there is any association between miR ratio and tumor size in patients ($N = 271$). Data were also collected on tumor grade, presence of lymphovascular invasion, presence of metastasis to axillary lymph nodes, and hormone receptor status. No matching was done. Exploratory analyses showed that miR ratio is normally distributed, also supported by the quantile-quantile (Q-Q) plot which shows that the quantiles of the observed data set (y-axis) follow a fairly tight straight line along the theoretical quantiles of normal distribution (x-axis) (Figure 5.8) (**see online materials; available at www.demosmedical.com/pathology-data-sets**). All variables except miR ratio and tumor size are categorically coded.

How should we assess the association? A summary of tumor characteristics is given in Table 5.3. A two-way scatter plot suggests a positive linear relationship between tumor size and level of miR ratio in blood (Figure 5.9). Pearson correlation coefficient is 0.99. In order to further quantify the association, we may fit the data with a general linear regression model.

Fitting and interpreting the model: No collinearity is detected among predictors given the low VIF values (Figure 5.10). We then run a univariable model separately for each predictor with the command **regress miR_ ratio Tumor_size** (and then do the same for all variables). It turns out that only lymph node metastasis and tumor size are statistically significantly associated with the level of miR ratio. Let's take a closer look at the univariable regression output for the association between tumor size and miR ratio (Figure 5.11A). The output suggests that the regression model explains 97.5% of the variability of miR ratio in the sample (as indicated by the R-squared value) and in the population (as given by the adjusted

(text continues on page 109)

TABLE 5.3
Tumor Characteristics in Study Population (*N* = 271; Hypothetical Data)

TUMOR CHARACTERISTICS	TOTAL *N* = 271 *n* (col %)
Tumor size (cm)	Mean: 4.97 SD: 0.93
miR ratio	Mean: 0.45 SD: 0.18
Tumor grade	
Well differentiated	54 (20)
Moderately differentiated	164 (61)
Poorly differentiated	53 (19)
Metastasis	
No	128 (47)
Yes	143 (53)
Presence of lymphovascular invasion	
No	229 (85)
Yes	42 (15)
Hormone receptor status	
ER+/PR+	118 (44)
ER+/PR–	96 (35)
ER–/PR+	23 (8)
ER–/PR–	34 (13)

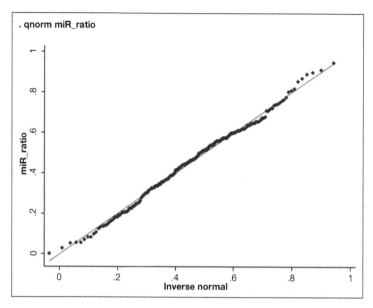

FIGURE 5.8
Q-Q plot of miR ratios in the data set against theoretical quantiles of normal distribution.

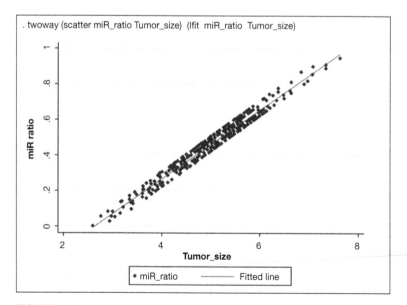

FIGURE 5.9
Two-way scatter plot on the association of miR ratio with tumor size.

```
. xi: quietly regress  miR_ratio Tumor_size Metastasis LVI  i.Tumor_grade i.Receptor
i.Tumor_grade      _ITumor_gra_0-2    (naturally coded; _ITumor_gra_0 omitted)
i.Receptor         _IReceptor_0-3     (naturally coded; _IReceptor_0 omitted)

. vif
```

Variable	VIF	1/VIF
_ITumor_gr~2	2.23	0.448054
_ITumor_gr~1	1.83	0.545917
Metastasis	1.72	0.580485
Tumor_size	1.64	0.608229
_IReceptor_3	1.46	0.686964
_IReceptor_1	1.36	0.736515
_IReceptor_2	1.16	0.859100
LVI	1.09	0.914352
Mean VIF	1.56	

FIGURE 5.10
Checking for collinearity among variables.

A . regress miR_ratio Tumor_size

Source	SS	df	MS		
Model	8.7229867	1	8.7229867	Number of obs =	271
Residual	.227134216	269	.000844365	F(1, 269) =10330.82	
				Prob > F =	0.0000
				R-squared =	0.9746
				Adj R-squared =	0.9745
Total	8.95012092	270	.033148596	Root MSE =	.02906

miR_ratio	Coef.	Std. Err.	t	P>|t|	[95% Conf. Interval]
Tumor_size	.1938878	.0019076	101.64	0.000	.1901321 .1976435
_cons	-.5096387	.0096439	-52.85	0.000	-.5286259 -.4906516

B . xi: sw regress miR_ratio Tumor_size Metastasis LVI i.Tumor_grade i.Receptor, pr(0.05)
```
i.Tumor_grade      _ITumor_gra_0-2    (naturally coded; _ITumor_gra_0 omitted)
i.Receptor         _IReceptor_0-3     (naturally coded; _IReceptor_0 omitted)
                   begin with full model
p = 0.7360 >= 0.0500  removing _IReceptor_3
p = 0.7148 >= 0.0500  removing _ITumor_gra_2
p = 0.5577 >= 0.0500  removing _IReceptor_1
p = 0.5310 >= 0.0500  removing _IReceptor_2
p = 0.2306 >= 0.0500  removing _ITumor_gra_1
p = 0.2099 >= 0.0500  removing LVI
```

Source	SS	df	MS		
Model	8.72802832	2	4.36401416	Number of obs =	271
Residual	.222092593	268	.000828704	F(2, 268) =	5266.07
				Prob > F =	0.0000
				R-squared =	0.9752
				Adj R-squared =	0.9750
Total	8.95012092	270	.033148596	Root MSE =	.02879

miR_ratio	Coef.	Std. Err.	t	P>|t|	[95% Conf. Interval]
Tumor_size	.1905025	.0023356	81.56	0.000	.185904 .195101
Metastasis	.0106778	.0043291	2.47	0.014	.0021545 .0192011
_cons	-.4984476	.0105767	-47.13	0.000	-.5192716 -.4776236

FIGURE 5.11
(A) Univariable model and (B) multivariable model (with backward selection) on the association between miR ratio and tumor size.

R-squared value). The unadjusted regression coefficient represents the amount of miR ratio increase associated with each 1 cm increase of tumor size (Figure 5.11A). Including the variable of nodal metastasis in the model does not significantly change the regression coefficient of tumor size (Figure 5.11B). The multivariable model output shows that after controlling for the presence of nodal metastasis, each 1 cm increase of tumor size is associated with 0.19 unit increase of miR ratio (95% CI: 0.19–0.20), and presence of nodal metastasis is associated with 0.01 unit increase of miR ratio after controlling for tumor size (95% CI: 0.002–0.192) (Figure 5.11B). Recall our discussion of predictor selection. The same principles and considerations apply here to decide on the final model. For general linear regression, a model-fit measure, the Akaike information criterion (AIC) (–2 * maximum log-likelihood) + (2 * # of parameters in the model) is one tool that can help to select the most parsimonious model, which has the lowest AIC value.

Regression diagnostics: Multiple methods are available from statistical packages to run diagnostics for general linear regression, including methods (a) to check for outlier and influential data, (b) to test for normality of residuals (deviations of the model predicted values from the observed values), and (c) to check for homoscedasticity (constant error variance). Details of regression diagnostics are readily available in books and online tutorials, for which selected advanced reading options are provided as references (12,13).

CAVEATS

What if our outcome variable is not normally distributed? Chapter 3 covers common methods to transform data to attain normality. When those methods fail, other models should be considered to fit the data.

What if the association of interest is not linear? The model can be modified to some extent to fit other functions. For example: Splines can be created to accommodate "knots" in the line to allow variation of slopes with different values of the independent variable (14).

What if the observations are correlated? This is common in longitudinal studies and clustered designs in which we get more than one measurement from the same patient. Models allowing assessment of random effects, such as generalized linear mixed models, would be needed to account for the correlations in the model.

TAKE-HOME POINTS

- Regression methods allow us to quantify the strength of the association of interest and to control for confounding and interaction by including multiple predictors in one model.
- Model fitting requires one to check for model assumptions, perform univariable and multivariable regression analyses, and assess how well the model fits the data.
- Predictor selection should be based on both research literature and statistical considerations.
- Understand the different assumptions and effect measures associated with commonly used regression models.
- Know how to interpret the regression outputs of logistic and linear regression models.

QUESTIONS FOR SELF-STUDY

1. Consider a hypothetical study: A research group wanted to investigate the effect of a new drug they developed on ovarian serous carcinoma in mouse models by measuring their tumor size after two groups of mice (*n* = 24 in each group) finished the regimen by intravenous (IV) or intraperitoneal drug therapies, respectively. They plotted the tumor sizes by drug dosage according to the route of drug administration (Figure 5.12).

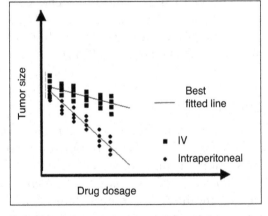

FIGURE 5.12
Scatter plots on the relationship between tumor size and drug dosage by drug administration (intravenous [IV] vs. intraperitoneal).

Based on the figure, how would you describe the relationship between tumor size and drug dosage? What effect does route of drug administration have on the association?

2. A study was presented on the relationship between alcohol consumption and colorectal cancer. Covariates included in the researchers' regression model were age, gender, smoking, folate intake, presence of comorbidities including diabetes and obesity, and physical activity. Peers criticized their analysis, stating that folate intake should not be included in the model because it was not statistically associated with colorectal cancer in the study population. Which one of the following responses would be appropriate to justify keeping folate intake in the model?

A. Folate intake was included because it may mediate the association between alcohol consumption and colorectal cancer.

B. Folate intake was included because of noncollapsibility in the statistical model.

C. Folate intake was correlated with alcohol consumption in the study population.

D. Folate intake was specified as a confounder a priori based on previous study findings.

E. There is no reason to keep folate intake in the model if it was not statistically significantly associated with the primary outcome in the study population.

Questions 3 and 4 are based on the following hypothetical study:

A group of researchers wanted to do a cross-sectional study to see whether parity was associated with breastfeeding in postpartum women in South Africa. Data on parity were collected as the number of previous births. Data on breastfeeding of the newborn were collected as a binary variable ("yes" or "no"). Other demographic data collected included women's age, educational status, marital status, family income, comorbidities, as well as age and number of current newborn.

3. The researchers decided to fit the data with a logistic regression model. Which of the following is true?

A. The researchers should interpret the effect measure of the statistical model as prevalence ratio.

B. The researchers should interpret the effect measure of the statistical model as OR.

C. The researchers should be aware that the OR yielded by the model can be an underestimate of the true prevalence ratio.

D. The researchers *must* fit the data with a GLM.

E. The researchers *never* fit such data with a logistic regression model.

4. In order to check whether it would be appropriate to fit the model with parity coded as a continuous variable, the researchers could:

A. Code parity as a categorical variable and fit a model with this variable. If the OR is significant, use parity as a continuous variable.

B. Fit models with backward stepwise selection of covariates and choose the model with the lowest AIC.

C. Fit a logistic model with dummy variables of parity so as to determine whether the change in log odds per previous birth is approximately linear. If so, use parity as a continuous variable.

D. Not use a logistic regression model, as it does not allow for continuous variable(s).

E. Only use a linear regression model to do that.

ANSWERS TO QUESTIONS FOR SELF-STUDY

1. By eyeballing, we see that tumor size and drug dosage seem to follow an inverse linear relationship, as tumor size decreases with increasing drug dosage. Route of drug administration appears to be an effect modifier with IV administration diminishing the effect of the drug on tumor size reduction as compared to intraperitoneal administration. One way to further work on these observations would be to use a regression model to evaluate the association between drug dosage and tumor size, and to test for interaction between drug dosage and drug administration in the model. This will allow us to quantify and test for statistical significance of the association and effect of interaction. Tumor size is a continuous variable, and a linear regression model is an option, provided that the data fulfill the assumptions (see Table 5.1).

2. Answer: D. Variables in a regression model are selected based on not just statistical considerations but also previous literature and biologic plausibility. As such, B and C are not the most appropriate responses. A is incorrect as inclusion of a mediator in the relationship between the primary exposure and outcome in the model would lead to underestimation of the primary effect measure.

3. Answer: B. The measure of association yielded by a logistic regression model is OR (B), and not prevalence ratio (A). In a setting where the prevalence of the studied outcome is high, OR can be a strong overestimate, not underestimate (C), of the prevalence ratio (aka "relative risk"). Option E is incorrect as a logistic regression model is a common and valid model used in analyzing cross-sectional study data with binary outcome. There are alternative models to obtain prevalence ratios, for example, log-binomial regression (a GLM). There is nothing intrinsically wrong with the use of OR in this case, so option D is incorrect.

4. Answer: C. A logistic regression model can be fitted with exposure/explanatory covariates coded as continuous variables, so options D and E are incorrect. Creating dummy variables is a reasonable way to study the variation and linearity of log odds per 1 unit change of parity (i.e., per previous birth). Option A does not at all assess the use of parity as a continuous variable, and option B is to check the model for parsimony and not variable coding. Hence both A and B are incorrect.

■ REFERENCES

1. Zhang HH, Cheng G, Liu Y. Linear or nonlinear? Automatic structure discovery for partially linear models. *J Am Stat Assoc.* 2011;106(495):1099-1112.

2. Segal MR. Tree-structured methods for longitudinal data. *J Am Stat Assoc.* 1992;87(418):407-418.

3. Eubank RL, Kamboura EL, Kimb JT, et al. Estimation in partially linear models. *Comput Stat Data Anal.* 1998;29(1):27-34.

4. Nelder J, Wedderburn R. Generalized linear models. *J R Stat Soc Ser A.* 1972;135(3):370-384.

5. Hidalgo B, Goodman M. Multivariate or multivariable regression? *Am J Public Health.* 2013;103(1):39-40.

6. Samadder NJ, Curtin K, Tuohy TM, et al. Characteristics of missed or interval colorectal cancer and patient survival: a population-based study. *Gastroenterology.* 2014;146(4):950-960.

7. McNutt LA, Wu C, Xue X, Hafner JP. Estimating the relative risk in cohort studies and clinical trials of common outcomes. *Am J Epidemiol.* 2003;157(10):940-943.

8. Zou G. A modified Poisson regression approach to prospective studies with binary data. *Am J Epidemiol.* 2004;159(7):702-706.

9. Greenland S. Model-based estimation of relative risks and other epidemiologic measures in studies of common outcomes and in case-control studies. *Am J Epidemiol.* 2004;160:301-305.

10. Soresi M, Magliarisi C, Campagna P, et al. Usefulness of alpha-fetoprotein in the diagnosis of hepatocellular carcinoma. *Anticancer Res.* 2003;23(2C):1747-1753.

11. Chen W, Cai F, Zhang B, et al. The level of circulating miRNA-10b and miRNA-373 in detecting lymph node metastasis of breast cancer: potential biomarkers. *Tumour Biol.* 2013;34(1):455-462.

12. Mitchell MN. *Interpreting and Visualizing Regression Models Using Stata.* College Station, TX: Stata Press; 2012:30-34, chap 2.

13. Chen X, Ender PB, Mitchell M, Wells C. *Stata Web Books. Regression with Stata. Chapter 2—Regression Diagnostics.* Available at http://www.ats.ucla.edu/stat/stata/webbooks/reg/chapter2/statareg2.htm

14. Mitchell MN. *Interpreting and Visualizing Regression Models Using Stata.* College Station, TX: Stata Press; 2012:79-126, chap 4; 325-364.

CHAPTER 6

Count Data and the Poisson Distribution
Danny A. Milner Jr.

◼ INTRODUCTION

In Figure 6.1, we see some data from a set of rat experiments where rats with sepsis had mitoses counted from the germinal centers of lymph nodes versus controls. Considering the number of cells per section of a lymph node, mitoses are a relative rare event. Temperature is also recorded for the rats, and we can see it is precisely measured to two decimal places.

Note that the mean, standard deviation, and variance of the temperature look very different from the same measure for the mitoses counts. Specifically, the mean is equal to the variance in the mitosis data. Based on these values, we can see that the mitotic count satisfies criteria to be analyzed as "count data." What exactly does that mean?

One of the first things we learn as children is to count on our fingers (and maybe toes).

This easily allows us to get to any number between 1 and 20. Unfortunately, counting is more complicated than that in that zero (0) is a valid count (but where do you signify zero fingers?) and, of course, we can count infinitely beyond 20. Much later in our mathematical education, we are introduced to fractions and decimals such that everything becomes a little more exact. This concept dominates our medical education, and we feel that a number really cannot be accurate unless there are one or two decimal places after it. When we write our first manuscript, we consider reporting the age of our patients in group A as 23.45 years (that looks so exact!) but our brains only think about 23-year-olds. We report 23.45

		Temperature (°C)	Mitoses/10 hpf
Sepsis	Rat 1	38.86	12
	Rat 2	38.83	14
	Rat 3	39.17	13
	Rat 4	38.67	15
	Rat 5	39.00	10
	Rat 6	39.14	5
	Rat 7	39.00	6
	Rat 8	39.00	15
	Rat 9	38.00	16
	Rat 10	39.00	14
	Rat 11	38.67	13
	Rat 12	39.00	11
Mean		38.86	12.00
St Dev		0.30	3.49
Variance		0.10	12.18
Controls	Rat 13	36.84	6
	Rat 14	36.70	1
	Rat 15	36.53	6
	Rat 16	36.56	8
	Rat 17	36.83	7
	Rat 18	36.70	6
	Rat 19	36.37	5
	Rat 20	37.03	6
	Rat 21	36.58	8
	Rat 22	36.45	6
	Rat 23	36.70	8
	Rat 24	36.70	1
Mean		36.67	5.67
St Dev		0.18	2.39
Variance		0.03	5.70
		T-test	Poisson Test
Statistical Test		< 0.0001	< 0.0001

FIGURE 6.1
Septic rats versus control rats ($n = 24$) with temperature and mitoses/
10 hpf recorded.

because it is the average (total age/total number of subjects). We
might want to report their average temperature as 37.14°C (but the
thermometer provided only one decimal place). These types of overly
precise reports are all over the literature and mostly ignored despite the

fact that every chemistry and physics professor in college told us to report decimal places only to the level that they were accurately measured. But when we think of counting, it becomes even odder. Assume we have seven classrooms in the 11th grade at Morsedale High School with a total of 540 students. The average count of students per classroom is 77.1, 77.14, or 77.143 (depending on how precise you want to be). But note that this is number per something (a rate). Fractional data are allowed in the rate as long as the translated whole numbers (how many students in 10 classrooms = 771, not 771.4) are reported. Count data and the Poisson statistics that support the data are special examples of "counting" when numbers are too large for binominal proportion and too small for normal distribution, which probably represents one of the most common situations encountered in pathology. The methods were developed to allow for statistical calculations of rare events as are often encountered in pathology.

■ LET'S LEARN TO COUNT

There are many different types of data discussed previously. Count data, however, is a special case because we are cataloging discrete events over some relative point. For example, we count mitoses, lymphoblasts, and lymph nodes. We must count them as discrete numbers and report them as such to be accurate. However, we must also count them per something (high-power field, germinal center, and colonic segment), which is when fractional values of the counts are allowed.

Before we dive into a pathological example, let's think about something simple that we encounter on a daily basis. Assume we have an intersection of two roads with a traffic light in both directions and sidewalks all around. There is a bus stop bench on one corner. From the perspective of a person sitting on the bench, what can we observe? Cars moving in four different directions, people moving in four different directions on two sides of the street, number of red lights, buses that stop in front of the bench, and so on. For all of these items, we can count them. We might count and say 26. 26 what? 26 cars. What about 26 cars? 26 cars stopped at the red light while we sat at the bench. How long did we sit at the bench? 58 minutes. The value of 26 cars/58 min (or 0.45 cars/min) is a rate (lambda or λ), and the data we have collected are counting data, which follow a Poisson distribution if certain assumptions are met.

The Poisson distribution (Figure 6.2) is the unique properties of λ that allow for calculation of predicted events and comparison for statistical testing (1).

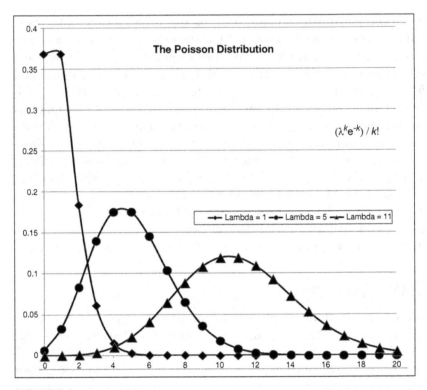

FIGURE 6.2
A graphical representation of the Poisson distribution given by the formula at the top right for a given mean (λ) and number of events (k).

The unique features include that the rate, λ, is also the variance. There are assumptions that must hold true for the Poisson distribution to fit data, which include (a) observations are whole number positive integers (i.e., discrete numbers from 0, 1, 2, 3, …); (b) all observations are independent; (c) the rate of observations is constant over the sample; (d) observations cannot occur at the same time; and (e) the probability of an observation is proportional to the length of the interval. Trying to use Poisson statistics if these assumptions do not hold true will result in an incorrect analysis. Let's look at our earlier example and see if this holds true.

We defined our observation as a car stopping at a red light. But we have to be more specific because for any given red light, there are two directions plus the number of lanes in each direction. If we specify the number of cars stopped going eastbound at a red light for a one-lane road, we are more accurately describing our events. But are we counting only the first car that is stopped or all cars that are stopped? One assumption for Poisson is that observations are independent. Clearly, the first car must stop because the light is red. All subsequent cars, however, must stop because the first car is stopped. So, to meet our assumptions, we would only be able to count the first car per red light. This also satisfies the assumption that the observations do not occur at the same time (only one car can be at the stop line in a single lane). We are also counting only whole cars (half cars tend to not drive very well) so our positive integer assumption is met. The last two assumptions are the most difficult. Does the rate of cars remain constant over the sample, and is the probability of seeing a car proportional to how long we watch? Imagine that we sat on the bus stop bench for 24 hours. We would observe that from midnight until 6 AM, the rate of cars would be highly variable (almost unpredictable). From 6 AM to 9 AM (or 4 PM to 7 PM) on a weekday (if our road is a commuting road), we'd likely see a steady rate of cars go through and the assumption might hold. Other times of the day, not so much. When we design a study where counting data will be measured, assuming the rate is constant or verifying this beforehand is important. Similarly, if our 58 minutes occurred after 6 AM as previously mentioned, we'd be comfortable with the last assumption of proportionality at least until 9 AM. After that, we cannot be sure this holds true. Imagine our other events mentioned and what different types of conditions we would have to apply to use Poisson statistics to evaluate our data.

Now let us consider a more practical pathology example. Consider 10 patients who have a core needle biopsy called malignant peripheral nerve sheath tumor (MPNST) for which you have counted mitoses in exactly 10-high-power fields for all cases. Because these are all MPNSTs (which we will assume have a mitosis definition of four or more per high-power field), one would estimate that there are at least 400 total mitoses in all patients in all cases counted ($4 \times 10 \times 10$) and that 100% of cases would have four or more mitoses per high-power field. The total number of mitoses is 563 (or 5.63 mitoses/high-power field per patient). A new experimental chemotherapy is given to all 10 patients and the tumor is resected. The same counts are repeated for a total of 236 mitoses (or 2.36 mitoses/high-power field per patient). Let us consider the components of each of these three situations (Table 6.1).

Lambda is the rate for each group expressed as a number (the right two columns in the table) and allows us to make comparisons between the groups using either the conditional test or C test (based on the null

TABLE 6.1
Comparisons of the Expected Versus Observed Counts by Different Field Types and λs

SAMPLE	TOTAL COUNT (k)	TOTAL FIELDS (n)	λ (TOTAL)	λ (PER PATIENT OR PER 10 HPF)
Definitional (expected)	400	100	4	40
Core needles (observed 1)	563	100	5.63	56.3
Status post chemotherapy (observed 2)	236	100	2.36	23.6

hypothesis that the ratio of λs is 1, less powerful) or the E test (based on the null hypothesis that the difference in λs = 0, more powerful) (2,3). In counting data, we know, based on the data, the direction of the effect and, thus, can use a one-tailed test for most Poisson calculations. If we plug the data for the per patient or per 10 hpf into a Poisson two-count calculator (freely available on the web) where we have an n of 10 (either 10 patients or 10 hpf) and λs of 56.3 and 23.6, we see that the P value for the C test is 0.0546 and the E test is < .0001. These are larger numbers and, in fact, the assumption of normality will hold true so we could just perform a t test of means. If we chose to use the "per high-power field per patient" numbers (5.63 and 2.36), we should use the Poisson tests.

When the counts are very small (two patients with cancer out of 25 patients who took drug A versus four patients with cancer out of 25 patients who took drug B) and reported as a proportion between 0 and 1, the assumptions for binomial distribution are met and we can use the binomial proportions test. Note also that these data would not meet the assumptions of Poisson as the rate of drug response is not necessarily predictable over the study. In simplest terms, the two proportions ($P_1 = 0.08$ and $P_2 = 0.16$) are compared over the sample size

(n = 25 per group) and a z-statistic for the binomial distribution is used to report a P value. The equation is given by:

$$\frac{P_1 - P_2}{\sqrt{(P_1)(1 - P_1)\,/\,n}}$$

For an alpha of 0.05, the z-statistic is evaluated for 1.96 $|z|$ > 1.96 to determine if the difference is significant (P value < .05).

When the numbers are very large or, better stated, not rare (500 patients out of 1,000 who smoked have peripheral vascular disease [PVD] vs. 100 patients out of 1,000 who did not smoke have peripheral vascular disease), the assumption of a normal distribution is met and parametric tests can be used. Note also that this data is not necessarily a rate that is predictable. For example, if we have 345 cars pass by the intersection of Fifth and Elm over a 2-hour period and 473 cars pass by the intersection of Eighth and Chestnut during the same 2-hour period, we could compare those numbers by a t test where the means are 172.5 and 236.5 (cars per hour), the standard deviations are 13.1 and 15.4 (square root of the variance = square root of the mean for Poisson data), and we have one observation of each, resulting in a P value of .00077. Similarly, larger tabulated data can be evaluated by the Fisher's exact test (smaller counts per cell) or chi-square test (larger counts per cell). In simplest terms for Fisher's exact test, the exact probability can be calculated as follows: $P = (a + b)!(c + d)!(a + c)!(b + d)!\,/\,a!b!c!d!n!$ from a two-by-two table of the form presented in Table 6.2.

In this example, the exact P value is <<< .0001 by Fisher's exact test. For chi-square, the equation is as follows:

$$\chi^2 = \Sigma\,(\text{observed value} - \text{expected value})^2/\text{expected value}$$

In this example, the chi-square value is 380.9 with 3° of freedom, and from a chi-square table the P value is <<< .0001. Remember that chi-square tests cannot be performed on tables if any individual cell has fewer than five counts per cell.

Poisson statistics are best used when the data fall between these somewhat rare events and the assumptions of the Poisson distribution are met.

Mitoses are counted as whole numbers and we do not, for example, count one half of a mitotic figure. Seeing a mitotic figure in one cell

TABLE 6.2
The Tabular Form of the Equation With the Numerical Example Included

	OUTCOME 1	OUTCOME 2			SMOKER	NONSMOKER	
Condition 1	a	b	$a + b$	PVD	500	100	600
Condition 2	c	d	$c + d$	No PVD	500	900	1,400
	$a + c$	$b + d$	$a + b + c + d = n$		1,000	1,000	2,000

does not mean we will see a mitotic figure in another cell and, more importantly, mitosis does not signal another cell to undergo mitosis (although some other external signal may be influencing the mitotic rate for a given tumor). If we divide a given tumor into 10 equal-sized squares, which contain, in each square, 10 high-power fields, we expect that we would get the same rate of mitoses in any given square as we do for any other given square. This assumption is the only one that may be problematic if, for example, mitoses are higher in one area of a tumor than in another (consider an area of fibrosarcomatous differentiation in a dermatofibrosarcoma protuberans). But our assumption is that, for the whole tumor, if we randomly sample, what we counted on one slide would be the same throughout. Hence, we are making this assumption. Otherwise, we would have to submit the entire sample and count every field. A cell can only contain a single mitosis so all events are discrete and one cannot count a single cell as two mitoses. Last, if we look at one field versus five fields versus 50 fields, the probability of seeing mitosis is expected to be the same and, thus, proportional to the number of fields we observe (otherwise, we would not be able to count only a limited number of fields!). That is, if we see one in three fields (0.33), we should see two in six fields, and we should see 20 in 60 fields.

Let us consider some examples of pathology data that would appear to be count data but for which each of the aforementioned assumptions would be violated, requiring different techniques. We may consider immunohistochemical staining for nuclei (or whole cells) as a yes/no event and, thus, be able to count them per high-power field, per total cells, and so forth. If we are scoring immunohistochemistry as 0, 1+, 2+, 3+ for a given stain, we now have a degree of uncertainty in whether an event is a "yes" or a "no" and it would cease to meet the whole number positive integer assumption. If we wanted to compare the relative rate of sodium performed in a day by an analyzer to another lab value, we would not be able to pick potassium as our comparator because the two tests are almost always ordered together in a panel and, thus, are not independent. In trying to plan our frozen section room budget, counting the number of frozen sections ordered by a surgical service over a 24-hour period would not meet the assumption that the rate of observations is constant, because of differences in operating room schedules and the days on which services operate. Similarly, if we observe the number of prostate biopsies we receive on a Tuesday and try to project numbers for the month, we may fail in the assumption that an equal number of biopsies are done every day (especially if Tuesday is "Prostate Biopsy Clinic Day"). When designing studies and evaluating the type of data that will be produced, a mental exercise of checking these assumptions is required to make sure Poisson approaches will hold.

When a data set contains a variable that is count data and it is the primary outcome we are interested in (assume we want to predict it), we can employ Poisson regression (a special type of regression) to get our values for the covariates of interest (4,5). This is true if our outcome is a rate and/or for certain types of survival analysis (6). Let us look at an example.

A set of 100 women age 35 to 75 who have either an abnormal ovarian ultrasound (oophrectomy with endometrial biopsy) or an normal ovary removed (as part of a hysterectomy) were studied to understand the relationship between endometrial stromal mitoses and ovarian pathology. Age, menopause status, parity, and number of mitoses in endometrial epithelial stroma in 100-high-power fields were collected. The goal was to understand what the effect on stromal mitoses were from all of these factors. A regression model would be the best approach to answer this question. In this case, however, the outcome variable (mitoses) meets the assumptions for Poisson counting data and, thus, Poisson regression is used. The output from Stata is shown in Figure 6.3.

The results demonstrate a full model (all variables, upper) with ovarian ultrasound abnormality being significantly associated with increasing mitotic rate while the other variables are not significant (note the P values and confidence intervals that contain 0). If we perform just the univariate model (as no other variables are significant in any iteration of the model), we see that the ultrasound variable remains with a strong association. Note the standard error is actually decreased in the univariate model (vs. the multivariate model) for ovarian ultrasound, suggesting that none of the other covariates are necessary to refine the coefficient estimate. A goodness-of-fit test for both models shows an excellent fit with or without covariates, suggesting that the association with increasing mitoses and abnormal ultrasounds is strong.

There are more assumptions with Poisson regression, including the challenge of overdispersion (where the variance is greater than the mean) and excessive zeros (more counts of zero than would be predicted by a Poisson distribution). If you need to employ Poisson regression and have questions, it is best to involve a statistician to make sure that model is appropriate or if alternative models are needed.

As with any evaluation of data, understanding the form of the data is crucial to proper analysis. In the special case of count data (that meets assumptions), which is common in pathological studies, the form of the

```
. poisson mitoses age menopause parity ovaryus

Iteration 0:     log likelihood = -210.31986
Iteration 1:     log likelihood = -210.31986

Poisson regression                          Number of obs    =        100
                                            LR chi2(4)       =      61.96
                                            Prob > chi2      =     0.0000
Log likelihood = -210.31986                 Pseudo R2        =     0.1284
```

mitoses	Coef.	Std. Err.	z	P>|z|	[95% Conf. Interval]	
age	.00406	.0059441	0.68	0.495	-.0075902	.0157102
menopause	.0289617	.1432666	0.20	0.840	-.2518357	.309759
parity	.004836	.0275643	0.18	0.861	-.0491891	.0588611
ovaryus	.6195525	.0822142	7.54	0.000	.4584157	.7806893
_cons	1.308078	.290281	4.51	0.000	.7391382	1.877019

```
. estat gof

          Goodness-of-fit chi2   =    53.72493
          Prob > chi2(95)        =     0.9998

. poisson mitoses ovaryus

Iteration 0:     log likelihood = -211.48847
Iteration 1:     log likelihood = -211.48847

Poisson regression                          Number of obs    =        100
                                            LR chi2(1)       =      59.63
                                            Prob > chi2      =     0.0000
Log likelihood = -211.48847                 Pseudo R2        =     0.1236
```

mitoses	Coef.	Std. Err.	z	P>|z|	[95% Conf. Interval]	
ovaryus	.6068687	.0800825	7.58	0.000	.4499098	.7638275
_cons	1.562185	.0635001	24.60	0.000	1.437727	1.686643

```
. estat gof

          Goodness-of-fit chi2   =    56.06214
          Prob > chi2(98)        =     0.9998
```

FIGURE 6.3
Output of two different Poisson regressions are shown for a full model (upper) and the reduced model (lower).

data can be easily recognized and the correct tests performed. When initially considering the design of a study, if the form of the data is not easily recognized, consultation with a statistician is key to appropriate data collection and testing.

TAKE-HOME POINTS

- When an experiment may result in the observation of rare events, consider Poisson statistics for comparisons or regressions.

- If a variable appears to be counting data, confirm that the assumptions of a Poisson data set are met.

- Binomial proportions testing, Poisson statistics, and Fisher's exact or chi-square test may all fit the form of a given data set but should not be used interchangeably; check the assumptions of each before beginning analysis.

QUESTIONS FOR SELF-STUDY

1. A new article in your favorite journal reports a finding that purports to predict high survivor rates in patients with acral lentiginous melanoma (ALM) based on an immunohistochemical stain for a novel protein counted in 10-high-power fields. The study collected 127 ALMs from eight different surgical centers and performed expression profiling to find the novel protein. A rabbit polyclonal antibody was generated to the protein from human tissue purification. The protein is highly expressed in bile duct epithelium, which was used as a control. The data in the paper shows that for the 34 patients who had greater than 5-year metastasis-free disease their tumors had a total of 500 positive cells. In the remaining 93 patients who had less than 5 years of metastasis-free disease their tumors had a total of 500 positive cells. What is the rate of tumor cells per patient in each group? Are the rates significantly different? (www.statstod.com/TwoCounts_Pgm.php may be helpful in answering these questions.)

2. A new junior partner in your pathology group wants to engage in a quality assurance/quality improvement project and asks you about evaluating your group's use of special stains for infections in-house versus sending cases for consultation. You report that infectious cases are pretty rare in your group but the project is worthwhile. Six months later, the junior partner returns with data and shows you the following table with statistics (E test):

CASE TYPE (TOTAL PER 6 MONTHS)	NO. OF SPECIAL STAINS ORDERED	NO. OF EXTERNAL CONSULTS	P VALUE
Breast (435)	16	7	< .001

(continued)

(*continued*)

CASE TYPE (TOTAL PER 6 MONTHS)	NO. OF SPECIAL STAINS ORDERED	NO. OF EXTERNAL CONSULTS	P VALUE
GI (652)	36	19	< .001
Skin (1101)	159	35	< .001

What are the primary issues with the way the data are reported?

3. A technical director (TD) in the chemistry laboratory brings to your attention a problem with barcode label positions on green top tubes that is causing a failure to read by the laboratory tracking system. The TD suspects that the problem is with nurse-drawn samples versus phlebotomist-drawn samples.

Data are extracted from the laboratory information system for a 24-hour period and presented as follows. Is the problem with labeling due to staff or shift?

DRAWN BY	SHIFT	NO. OF TUBES	NO. OF LABEL FAILS
Nurse	1st	42	2
Phlebotomist	1st	267	1
Nurse	2nd	36	2
Phlebotomist	2nd	346	2
Nurse	3rd	145	23
Phlebotomist	3rd	37	1

ANSWERS TO QUESTIONS FOR SELF-STUDY

1. The smaller group (34) has a rate of 14.7 positive cells per patient per 10-high-power field, and the larger group (93) has a rate of 5.4 positive cells per patient per 10-high-power field, and the difference is significant by the C and E tests of two Poisson counts.

2. In order to "count" the special stains versus the "consults," we have to meet the assumptions of the Poisson distribution to use the E test as reported. In this case, the special stain cases and the consult cases come from the same pool of patients (possibly from the same case) so they are not independent. Moreover, we do not have a way to objectively divide the 435 breast cases, for example, into those where we observe the use of a special stain versus those where we observe the use of a consult (we don't know the denominator). Last, a given case may need more than one special stain, which also does not satisfy the assumptions of occurring at the same time.

3. At first look, we might conclude that the third shift nurses are the issue. However, if we compare nurse to phlebotomist for all shifts, we see a significant difference indicating that nurses for all shifts are a problem. Most importantly, when we compare nurse to nurse for all shifts, we do not see a significant difference. Thus, nurse education about labels is the key to solving this problem.

■ REFERENCES

1. Haight F. *Handbook of the Poisson Distribution*. New York, NY: John Wiley & Sons; 1967.
2. Krishnamoorthy K, Thomson J. A more powerful test for comparing two Poisson means. *J Stat Plan Inference*. 2004;119:23-35.
3. Przyborowski J, Wilenski H. Homogeneity of results in testing samples from Poisson series. *Biometrika*. 1940;31:313-323.
4. Cameron A, Trivedi P. *Regression Analysis of Count Data*. Cambridge, United Kingdom: Cambridge University Press; 1998.
5. Meyer JE, Cohen SJ, Ruth KJ, et al. Young age increases risk of lymph node positivity in early-stage rectal cancer. *J Natl Cancer Inst*. 2016;108.
6. Raine-Bennett T, Tucker LY, Zaritsky E, et al. Occult uterine sarcoma and leiomyosarcoma: incidence of and survival associated with morcellation. *Obstet Gynecol*. 2016;127:29-39.

CHAPTER 7

Survival Analyses: Cox Proportional Hazards Model

T. Rinda Soong
Danny A. Milner Jr.

■ INTRODUCTION

In Chapter 5, we discussed how regression modeling helps define associations between predictors and events of interest in cross-sectional analyses. In this chapter, we highlight common approaches to analyzing time-to-event data. After defining functions and concepts related to survival analyses, we illustrate the application of the Cox proportional hazards model in the context of a motivating example. Validity of a model is briefly discussed in the last section.

Consider all of the following scenarios: the production of a harvestable fruit from a fruit tree, the presence of kidney failure in a diabetic patient, the failure of a brake pad to stop a car adequately, and the death of a person with a staged cancer. In each of these situations, we have an event that will occur or will not occur (picking a fruit, kidney failure, brake failure, death) which we monitor over a time period of observation. If we are looking at a single bud on a fruit tree, we can report a time (e.g., 3 months to produce a fruit). The same is true of a single patient (e.g., Mr. Jones developed kidney failure after 6 months). The important features here are that the observation has a start time and for each individual there is a "stop time" (time at which the event of interest occurs). If we have a large collection of individuals (fruits, patients, or brakes) that we can observe over the same time frame (not necessarily at the same time), plotting this data would produce a "time-to-event" curve.

This curve is purely descriptive and, in itself, may have value for making decisions. However, when we have other variables to consider, modeling survival data is needed to understand what affects the time to developing the event of interest for any given observation.

■ WHAT IS SURVIVAL ANALYSIS?

In many studies, the primary outcome of interest is the time to developing an event. Survival analysis (better thought of as "time-to-event" analysis) allows us to evaluate the association of predictors with the time to the event of interest, which can be death, disease recurrence, metastasis, complete remission, and so on. The time of origin (beginning of the time of observation), the time scale, and the event of interest need to be clearly defined for proper analysis. Common functions used to describe survival data include the following (1–3):

- **Survival function** at time t, $S(t)$: This is the probability of being event-free at time t (i.e., the probability that the survival time is greater than t).

- **Cumulative incidence function** at time t, $1 - S(t)$: This defines the probability that the event has occurred by time t.

- **Hazard function** at time t, $h(t)$: This is the instantaneous rate of event occurrence at time t given that the event has not occurred yet. For practical purposes, hazard may be roughly interpreted as the incidence rate, though they are not exactly the same (1). Hazard ratio (HR), which is the ratio of hazards of the exposed and unexposed groups to a predictor of interest, is a common effect measure in survival analysis. Since HR is time-dependent, differences seen with period-specific HRs may suggest introduction of selection bias in a prospective study or change in effect over time, and a single averaged HR reported over a study period can be potentially misleading. Hence, examining the survival curves adjusted for confounders is a helpful tool for analysis and HR interpretation.

■ CENSORING IN SURVIVAL STUDIES

Since subjects may enter and leave a study at different time points, it is often impossible to know when exactly the event of interest occurs for every individual in the study population. This phenomenon is called "censoring," which can be classified into three categories (4):

- **Right censoring:** This is the most common scenario of censoring. Subjects are followed for a period of time t in the study, and then they are no longer observed. This can happen for a number of reasons:

  - Subjects develop the event of interest at time t.

  - Subjects are lost to follow-up or they withdraw from the study.

  - The study ends and the event has not yet occurred for some subjects by that time.

- **Left censoring:** This arises when the event occurred before the subject enters the study. For example, a man enters a study examining factors influencing persistence of anal warts and is found to have a positive anal Pap smear and a small anal wart at baseline visit.

- **Interval censoring:** This can happen when a subject was lost to follow-up for a time interval during the study, and is then found to have developed the event when follow-up resumes. Consequently, we do not know the exact time point at which the event developed. Strictly speaking, all studies are subject to interval censoring, as follow-up happens at fixed time points and there is no way for us to ascertain when exactly between the follow-up time points the event occurred. Mathematically, interval censoring is the same as left censoring.

Caveats

INFORMATIVE VERSUS NONINFORMATIVE CENSORING

Survival analysis entails the assumption that censorship is noninformative; that is, the survival time of a subject is independent of a mechanism that would cause a subject to be censored. For instance, it is assumed in survival analysis that subjects who are censored at any time would have the same survival prospects as those who continue to be followed. Informative censoring introduces bias, and standard methods of survival analysis do not work well when that happens. Although different models and ad hoc sensitivity analysis have been proposed to approach situations with informative censoring (5), the best solution is always to minimize dropout via study design. Consider a 20-year study looking at time to development of adenocarcinoma in patients who have adenomas at first colonoscopy. If, during the 20 years, an alternative approach is put into use that includes total colectomy for patients with more than 10 adenomas at first colonoscopy (thus removing or censoring patients from our study), this would be informative censoring because it would affect the outcome as we would expect patients with more adenomas to have higher rates of cancer. In contrast, the loss of a fruit tree in a storm or the selling of a car for scrap is unrelated to the production of fruit or brake failure from use—thus, it is noninformative censoring.

CAUSE-SPECIFIC SURVIVAL AND COMPETING RISKS

Overall survival refers to time to an event, such as death, from any causes. Oftentimes studies are more interested in examining the cause-specific survival, which is time to an event from a specific cause. A subject may experience an event other than the one of interest and that alters the probability of experiencing the event of interest. These events are termed "competing events." One example would be cancer patients who are subject to developing various events, such as distant metastases, local recurrence, or death, which preclude development of other events (6,7). Applying standard survival analyses such as Kaplan–Meier (KM) estimator and taking other competing events as censored observations may be a biased approach (7). Appropriate methods, which have been described in literature, should be applied to obtain a correct estimate of the cumulative probability of each event, and influence of competing risks should be considered when comparing cause-specific outcomes between groups (6–9).

What Models Can We Use to Evaluate Survival Data and Predict the Survival Probabilities in the Population?

Linear and logistic regression models do not work with time-to-event data because they cannot take into account censoring and the different lengths of follow-up time in the analyses. Some common examples of survival models with covariates used for censored data are the following (2):

- Parametric families of distributions assume the survival functions follow a specific distribution. Examples of distributions include exponential, Weibull, generalized gamma, lognormal, log-logistic, or generalized F.

- Accelerated failure time models are parametric models which assume the predictor accelerates or decelerates the development of the event by a constant (10).

- Proportional hazards models are models which make the assumption of proportional hazards. We will go into greater detail about this model later in the chapter.

- Frailty models are random effects models for time variables where the random effects (frailty) have a multiplicative effect on the hazard. They are commonly used to model correlated failure time data (11).

We use the following example to illustrate the basic approach to analyzing survival data.

■ EXAMPLE: TUMOR GRADE AND SURVIVAL IN PATIENTS WITH COMPLETE RESPONSE TO NEOADJUVANT TREATMENT OF ESOPHAGEAL ADENOCARCINOMA

Heterogeneity in disease recurrence and 5-year survival has been observed in patients who had pathologic complete response to neoadjuvant treatment for esophageal adenocarcinoma. A study was performed to examine the clinicopathologic features associated with survival and disease recurrence in these patients (12). A data set was adapted from this study's parent data set for illustration. For the purpose of our discussion, we define death as our event of interest and assess the association of time to death (i.e., the overall survival) with the tumor grade (high vs. low) seen in pretreatment esophageal biopsy. Extent of sampling in the resection specimen posttreatment (incomplete vs. complete sampling of tumor bed) will be evaluated as a potential confounder as a practice example. How should we approach the data? (**See online materials; available at www.demosmedical.com/pathology-data-sets**).

Describe the Data

We can import the data into statistical software to do the analyses. Data outputs shown in this section are based on Stata using the commands **stset, stci, stir,** and **stsum,** assuming the data are of the proper format for survival data and that the time variable and event variable are defined. The commands function as follows: **stset** defines data as survival data; **stci** produces confidence intervals; **stir** reports incidence-rate comparison; and **stsum** summarizes the survival-time data. Both tumor grade and survival status are binary-coded in this example, with low-grade tumor and being alive as reference categories respectively. Output in Figure 7.1A shows how the command **stset** sets up the survival data by designating "Days_to_Death" as the time variable in relation to the event of interest (i.e., "**Death**") by each subject (i.e., "**Case**"). The output shows that we have 93 patients in this data set, of whom 57 died during the study period. The median follow-up time was 1,734 days (57.8 months) in the total study population (Figure 7.1B). Fifty-one subjects had high-grade tumors in pretreatment biopsies, of whom 36 died during follow-up (Figure 7.2A). The incidence rate of death among them is twofold higher than those with low-grade tumors (incidence rate ratio = 2.0; 95% CI: 1.13–3.60) (Figure 7.2B). Patients with high-grade tumors had a lower median survival time (34.4 months, i.e., 1,032 days) than those with low-grade tumors

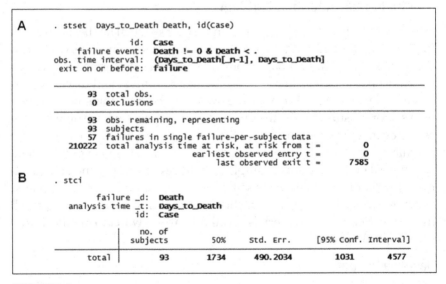

FIGURE 7.1
Brief description of survival data.

```
A    . stir  Tumor_grade_bin

           failure _d:  Death
     analysis time _t:  Days_to_Death
                   id:  case

     note:  Exposed <-> Tumor_grade_bin==High and unexposed <-> Tumor_grade_bin==Low

                          Tumor_grade_bin
                        Exposed   unexposed        Total

            Failure         36          21           57
               Time      97176      113046       210222

     Incidence Rate     .0003705    .0001858     .0002711

                        Point estimate          [95% conf. Interval]

     Inc. rate diff.       .0001847     .0000399    .0003295
     Inc. rate ratio      1.994249     1.133214    3.595311  (exact)
     Attr. frac. ex.      .4985581      .117554    .7218599  (exact)
     Attr. frac. pop      .3148788

                      (midp)   Pr(k>=36) =              0.0055  (exact)
                      (midp) 2*Pr(k>=36) =              0.0110  (exact)


B    . stsum, by (Tumor_grade_bin)

           failure _d:  Death
     analysis time _t:  Days_to_Death

                                  incidence      no. of   |——— survival time ———|
     Tumor_~n | time at risk        rate       subjects    25%      50%      75%

          Low |      113046       .0001858          42     974     3042       .
         High |       97176       .0003705          51     350     1032     5696

        total |      210222       .0002711          93     590     1734     5900
```

FIGURE 7.2

Comparison of incidence rate ratios between patients with high-grade tumors versus patients without low-grade tumors.

(median survival time: 101.4 months, i.e., 3,042 days) (Figure 7.2B). These findings suggest that subjects with high-grade tumors might have a poorer overall survival rate than those with low-grade tumors. Let's do more analyses to compare their time-to-death data.

Examine the Survival Curves by Kaplan–Meier Estimates

We can take a closer look at the subjects' respective survival functions with the use of Kaplan–Meier (KM) estimates, which give nonparametric estimates of the probabilities of surviving in a given length of time while considering time in small intervals. Subjects who have died or dropped out of the study are not counted as at risk and are considered censored. Figure 7.3A shows the KM survival curves of those who had high-grade tumors versus those who had low-grade tumors.

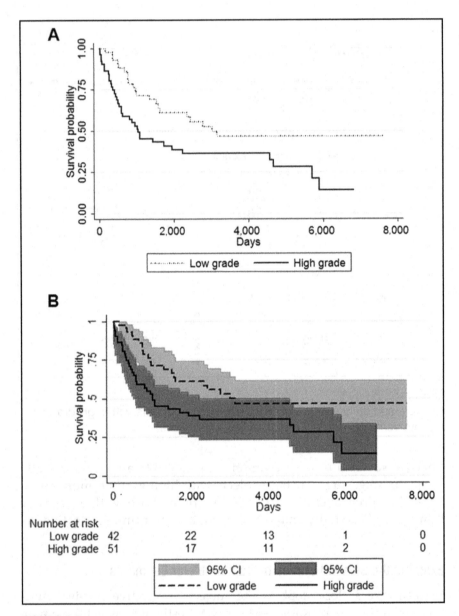

FIGURE 7.3
Kaplan–Meier survival curves by tumor grade.

Caveat

DISPLAYING KAPLAN–MEIER CURVES

The graph in Figure 7.3A is short of certain information that should be included (13):

- Extent of follow-up during the study: This can be shown by listing the number at risk at regular intervals under the time axis.

- Measures of statistical uncertainty: e.g., Standard errors or confidence intervals can be displayed at regular time points.

Figure 7.3B shows more informative KM curves enriched with the data listed earlier. Suppose we have a very low event rate in our study population, e.g., less than 30% of subjects develop the event, then we may consider displaying the graph "upward," i.e., showing the cumulative incidence percentage (in a range of 1%–30% or a smaller range if appropriate) instead of the survival probability (in a range of 1%–100%) in the y-axis (13). The advantage is that it can maximize the clarity of any difference in curves. If we display the curves "downward," then any differences in the curves would be hard to visualize because of the low event rate. An alternative would be to create a break in the vertical axis of the survival probability, but that break needs to be clear on the graph to avoid creating any misleading impression of a big difference between curves.

Let's look at the KM curves more closely in this example. By eyeballing, our curves appear to show that those who had high-grade tumors did worse than those who had low-grade tumors. We can do a total curve comparison by the log-rank test using the command **sts test** with the option **logrank**. Using the help function in Stata with "**sts test**" will give you a complete list of options as well as the form of the command. This is a test applicable for two or more survival functions. It tests the null hypothesis that there is no difference between the groups in the survival probabilities at each follow-up time. The test output in Figure 7.4 confirms that we can reject the null hypothesis ($P = .02$). KM analyses adjusted for confounder are feasible with statistical packages.

It should be noted, however, that if there is crossing of survival curves during the study, then the test does not work well as it tests

Log-rank test for equality of survivor functions		
Tumor_grad~n	Events observed	Events expected
Low	21	29.73
High	36	27.27
Total	57	57.00
	chi2(1) =	5.40
	Pr>chi2 =	0.0201

FIGURE 7.4
Log-rank test comparing survival functions between patients with high-grade tumors and patients with low-grade tumors.

the overall survival functions. Furthermore, KM estimates and log-rank test are limited to analyses with categorical predictors, and cannot accommodate continuous variables or time-dependent variables, for which a statistical model would be required for analyses.

Evaluate the Association by Fitting a Model

A model allows us to quantify the association of interest, to adjust the effect estimate for confounding, and to check for interactions among predictors in the model, the latter of which is difficult to do with adjusted KM estimates or stratified analyses, particularly when there are multiple predictors involved in the causal pathway of interest. The Cox proportional hazards model is a semi-parametric model and is by far the most commonly used model in survival studies. The effect estimate given by the model is the HR. In the Cox model, no assumption is made for the form of the *baseline* hazard (the nonparametric component of an otherwise parametric model), but it assumes that the HR is constant across time, and that the predictors act multiplicatively on hazards. In other words, proportional hazards are assumed over time. Since testing for proportionality of hazards in the data set requires calculation of the residuals, which are differences between the observed values in the sample and the predicted values based on the model, we need to first fit a Cox model before we can verify whether the assumption is met.

Fitting a Cox Proportional Hazards Model

In Chapter 5, we went over the basic steps in fitting logistic and linear regression models. The same principles apply to fitting a Cox model: first we need to run univariable analyses with each predictor, and then perform predictor selection and test for interactions to come up with a final model. Both tumor grade (binary variable: "**Tumor_grade_bin**") and completeness of tumor bed sampling (binary variable: "**Incomplete**") were found to be statistically significantly associated with the time to death in univariable analyses. We can check if keeping both variables in the model contribute to a better data fit with the likelihood ratio test, which involves fitting a restricted model (with only tumor grade as a single predictor) (Figure 7.5A), and then comparing it with an extended model (with both tumor grade and completeness of tumor bed sampling in the model) (Figure 7.5B). The likelihood ratio test assesses the null hypothesis that the models fit the data equally well. Based on the output of the likelihood ratio test (Figure 7.5B), we can reject the null hypothesis ($P = .0004$) and will keep both variables in the model.

Note that the HR associated with tumor grade, our primary predictor of interest, does not change significantly before and after adding the variable of sampling to the model. According to the output data, we conclude that patients who had high-grade tumor in their pretreatment biopsies have close to 2-fold increased hazard of death after controlling for completeness of tumor bed sampling (adjusted HR: 1.90; 95% CI: 1.10–3.26). Incomplete sampling of the tumor bed is associated with a 2.6-fold increased hazard of death after adjusting for tumor grade in the pretreatment biopsy (adjusted HR: 2.61; 95% CI: 1.52–4.47) (Figure 7.5B). Figure 7.6 shows that an interaction term ("**sample_grade**") added between tumor grade and tumor bed sampling in the model is not associated with a statistically significant effect estimate (HR: 0.97; 95% CI: 0.32–2.94). The results suggest that there is no interaction between the two variables in predicting time to death.

What If We Have Tied Events in Our Data Set?

Tied events are events having exactly the same survival times. It matters because the Cox model specifies a partial likelihood function, which

```
A    . stcox Tumor_grade_bin, nolog

           failure _d: Death
        analysis time _t: Days_to_Death

     Cox regression -- no ties

     No. of subjects =        93          Number of obs   =        93
     No. of failures =        57
     Time at risk    =    210222
                                          LR chi2(1)      =      5.44
     Log likelihood =  -225.46484         Prob > chi2     =    0.0197

     _t  | Haz. Ratio  Std. Err.    z    P>|z|    [95% Conf. Interval]

     Tumor_grad~n |  1.87839   .5177103  2.29   0.022   1.094417   3.223953

     . estimates store m1

B    . stcox Tumor_grade_bin Incomplete, nolog

           failure _d: Death
        analysis time _t: Days_to_Death

     Cox regression -- no ties

     No. of subjects =        93          Number of obs   =        93
     No. of failures =        57
     Time at risk    =    210222
                                          LR chi2(2)      =     18.09
     Log likelihood =  -219.13756         Prob > chi2     =    0.0001

     _t  | Haz. Ratio  Std. Err.    z    P>|z|    [95% Conf. Interval]

     Tumor_grad~n |  1.895863  .5231796  2.32   0.020   1.103851   3.256142
     Incomplete~g |  2.609115  .7156524  3.50   0.000   1.524115   4.466514

     . lrtest . m1

     Likelihood-ratio test                LR chi2(1)  =     12.65
     (Assumption: m1 nested in .)         Prob > chi2 =    0.0004
```

FIGURE 7.5
Likelihood ratio test comparing (A) univariable model with tumor grade
as a single predictor and (B) extended model with both tumor grade and
completeness of tumor bed sampling as predictor variables.

assumes that there are no tied events among the observations. In our
example with a relatively small sample size, there is no tied event as
noted in the model outputs. In real practice, time is usually measured
at discrete time points; hence, tied events are prone to occur. Several
methods have been developed to manage tied events. In general, when
we have large data sets or a large number of ties, Breslow's and Efron's
approximations might be used. When estimation precision is important, exact methods like exact marginal-likelihood method and exact
partial-likelihood method should be considered as they provide more
efficient parameter estimates (4).

```
. gen sample_grade= Incomplete_sampling*Tumor_grade_bin

. stcox Tumor_grade_bin Incomplete_sampling sample_grade, nolog

       failure _d: Death
   analysis time _t: Days_to_Death

Cox regression -- no ties

No. of subjects =          93          Number of obs    =        93
No. of failures =          57
Time at risk    =      210222
                                       LR chi2(3)       =     18.10
Log likelihood  =    -219.1363         Prob > chi2      =    0.0004
```

_t	Haz. Ratio	Std. Err.	z	P>|z|	[95% Conf. Interval]	
Tumor_grad~n	1.929186	.8557242	1.48	0.139	.8087398	4.601924
Incomplete~g	2.656214	1.194765	2.17	0.030	1.1	6.414067
sample_grade	.9719843	.5496617	-0.05	0.960	.3208491	2.944542

FIGURE 7.6
Check for interaction between tumor grade and completeness of tumor bed sampling.

How to Verify the Assumption of Proportional Hazards?

After we have fitted the Cox model, we can assess the data for the assumption of proportional hazards. One option is to perform a Schoenfeld test, which fits a linear regression model with time as the predictor and the scaled Schoenfeld residuals as the outcome. There is a Schoenfeld residual for each individual for each covariate, which is calculated as the difference between the observed value and the expected value assuming the hypotheses of the model are true. Figure 7.7A illustrates the Schoenfeld test output for the individual predictors. The correlation coefficient (rho) should be zero if the assumption holds and the P value needs to be less than .05 in order to reject the null hypothesis that the correlation is zero. According to the output for tumor grade, we cannot reject the null hypothesis and we believe the HR associated with tumor grade is constant (Figure 7.7A). The plot of the log–log transformation of the survival function versus time by tumor grade also shows two roughly parallel lines (Figure 7.7B), supporting the observation of proportional hazards.

Caveats

PROPORTIONAL VERSUS NONPROPORTIONAL HAZARDS

The Schoenfeld test output suggests that incomplete tumor bed sampling may be associated with an inconstant HR given that the

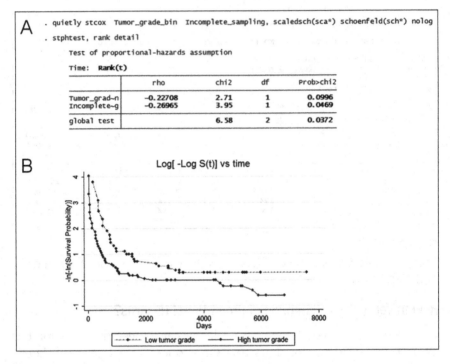

FIGURE 7.7
(A) Schoenfeld test on the model with tumor grade and completeness of tumor bed sampling as variables. (B) Log–log transformation of the survival function versus time by tumor grade.

P value for rho is less than .05. We can check on this by stratifying the Cox model by this variable. If it truly violates the assumption of proportionality, the estimates in the different strata would differ. In our example, the HR estimates associated with tumor grade in the strata of completeness of tumor sampling (1.90 and 1.84; Figure 7.8) are very similar to the HR estimate (1.896; Figure 7.5B) obtained from the model including tumor bed sampling as a predictor. This indicates that the hazards associated with tumor bed sampling are likely proportional. Another option is to include time-dependent covariates to assess for interactions of the predictors and time. The proportionality assumption is violated for that specific predictor if a time-dependent covariate is statistically significant.

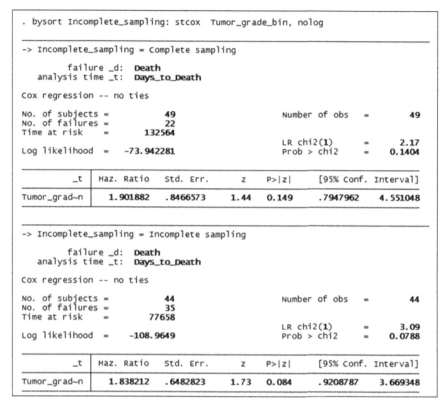

FIGURE 7.8
Stratified Cox analysis by the variable of tumor bed sampling.

WHAT IF THE PROPORTIONALITY ASSUMPTION OF HAZARDS IS TRULY VIOLATED?

We can modify the Cox model by adding time interaction terms, or we can apply a parametric model instead without assuming a constant HR, e.g., an accelerated failure time model, or other parametric survival models if the data fit a specific distribution.

WHAT IF EVENTS OF INTEREST ARE RECURRENT?

Some examples of recurrent events include cancer recurrence, sepsis, malaria episodes, positive human papillomavirus (HPV) test, positive Pap smear, and so on. Several modeling approaches have been proposed to account for the intra-subject correlation that arises from recurrent events in survival analysis and are available in different statistical packages (14).

How Can We Assess Goodness-of-Fit and Predictive Power of the Model?

One option is to use the Cox–Snell residuals to assess the overall fit of the model, which is readily available in statistical packages (15,16). Harrell's C and Somers' D statistics, for example, can be easily applied with statistical software to evaluate the predictive power of a survival model (17).

■ VALIDITY OF A MODEL

A good model is expected to give predicted probabilities closely matching those of the observed data (i.e., showing good calibration), and be able to distinguish lower- and higher-risk patients (i.e., having good discrimination) (5). A model that closely predicts the survival patterns of observed data is internally valid and can then be applied to clinical practice if its external validity (i.e., generalizability) can be validated. In a review done by Mallett et al. on the methodologies and reporting performance of 47 studies of prognostic models, it was found that a significant proportion of published prognostic models have been developed with poor methods and inadequate reporting information (18). Altman et al. discusses general approaches to validation with illustration of several case examples (19). Methods of external validation of published Cox model have also been proposed in literature for advanced reading and reference in practice (20,21).

TAKE-HOME POINTS

- The time of origin, the time scale, and the event of interest need to be unambiguously defined in survival analyses.
- Know the definitions of hazards and hazard ratio.
- Noninformative censoring is a basic and important assumption of all types of survival models.
- Choice of survival model depends on the distribution of the survival data and the research question.
- Know how to evaluate KM curves and know their limitations in assessing survival functions.
- Be familiar with the assumption and basic steps in fitting a Cox proportional hazards model.

- The internal validity and external validity of a prognostic model need to be validated before it can be generalized to clinical use.

QUESTIONS FOR SELF-STUDY

1. Define in words hazard function and censoring.
2. What is the most important underlying assumption of survival analyses?
3. Which of the following are the limitations of using KM estimate to assess survival functions (choose all that apply)?

    A. No adjustment, for example, confounder, can be made to the KM estimate.

    B. It can only be applied to comparison by a categorical variable.

    C. It cannot be applied to a continuous predictor variable.

    D. It is not appropriate for time-dependent variables.

4. A study was done to investigate the effect of tumor-receptor status and other covariates on mortality of patients diagnosed with breast cancer. Time-to-death data were collected. One may argue against the use of the conventional Cox proportional hazards regression model in such analysis because:

    A. Some covariates are time-dependent.

    B. The hazard rates may vary over time.

    C. Part of the data may be censored.

    D. The effect of exposure/covariate on mortality may not be constant over time in the study population.

    E. Cox regression model is not used for survival analysis.

5. Which of the following best describes the null hypothesis addressed by a log-rank test?

    A. No difference between the groups in the survival probabilities for at least one follow-up time.

    B. No difference between the groups in the proportion remaining at risk at each follow-up time.

    C. No difference between the groups in mean times-to-events.

D. No difference between the groups in the survival probabilities at each follow-up time.

E. No difference between groups in the proportion censored.

ANSWERS TO QUESTIONS FOR SELF-STUDY

1. Hazard function at time t, $h(t)$ is the instantaneous rate of event occurrence at time t (given that the event has not occurred yet).

   Censoring is a condition in which the value of a measurement or observation is only partially known.

2. The most important underlying assumption of survival analyses is that censorship is noninformative.

3. Answer: B, C, and D are the limitations of using KM estimate in assessing survival functions.

   Choice A is false because an adjustment, e.g., for confounding, can be made to the KM estimates and survival curve.

4. Answer: D. The Cox proportional hazards model is a statistical model used in survival analysis with hazard ratio being the effect measure of risk. The major assumption is that of proportional hazards; that is, the relative hazard of event in risk groups is constant at each follow-up time point. The assumption does not hold in this case as hazard ratio of death varies over time in patient groups with different tumor receptor status (22). Hazard rate (choice B) does not need to be constant, and covariates (choice D) themselves can be time-dependent in Cox regression analysis. Censoring (choice C) does not argue against the use of Cox regression model in this case.

5. Answer: D. A log-rank test is used to test the null hypothesis that the survival functions of the groups are the same at all follow-up times (23).

◼ REFERENCES

1. Hernán MA. The hazards of hazard ratios. *Epidemiology*. 2010; 21(1):13-15.

2. Bradburn MJ, Clark TG, Love SB, et al. Survival analysis part II: multivariate data analysis—an introduction to concepts and methods. *Br J Cancer*. 2003;89(3):431-436.

3. Bradburn MJ, Clark TG, Love SB, et al. Survival analysis Part III: multivariate data analysis—choosing a model and assessing its adequacy and fit. *Br J Cancer.* 2003;89(4):605-611.

4. Cleves M, Gould WW, Gutierrez RG, et al. *An Introduction to Survival Analysis Using Stata.* 2nd ed. College Station, TX: Stata Press; 2008.

5. Clark TG, Bradburn MJ, Love SB, et al. Survival analysis part IV: further concepts and methods in survival analysis. *Br J Cancer.* 2003;89(5):781-786.

6. Dignam JJ, Zhang Q, Kocherginsky M. The use and interpretation of competing risks regression models. *Clin Cancer Res.* 2012;18(8):2301-2308.

7. Andersen PK, Geskus RB, de Witte T, et al. Competing risks in epidemiology: possibilities and pitfalls. *Int J Epidemiol.* 2012;41(3):861-870.

8. Kim HT. Cumulative incidence in competing risks data and competing risks regression analysis. *Clin Cancer Res.* 2007;13(2 pt 1):559-565.

9. Satagopan JM, Ben-Porat L, Berwick M, et al. A note on competing risks in survival data analysis. *Br J Cancer.* 2004;91(7):1229-1235.

10. Hougaard P. Fundamentals of survival data. *Biometrics.* 1999; 55(1):13-22.

11. Hougaard P. Frailty models for survival data. *Lifetime Data Anal.* 1995;1(3):255-273.

12. Agoston AT, Zheng Y, Bueno R, et al. Predictors of disease recurrence and survival in esophageal adenocarcinomas with complete response to neoadjuvant therapy. *Am J Surg Pathol.* 2015;39(8):1085-1092.

13. Pocock, SJ, Clayton, TC, Altman, DG. Survival plots of time-to-event outcomes in clinical trials: good practice and pitfalls. *Lancet.* 2002;359:1686-1689.

14. Amorim LD, Cai J. Modeling recurrent events: a tutorial for analysis in epidemiology. *Int J Epidemiol.* 2015;44(1):324-333.

15. Stata survival analysis and epidemiological tables reference manual release 13. pp. 179-180. Available at http://www.stata.com/manuals13/st.pdf

16. R Package. *Survival analysis.* Available at: https://cran.r-project.org/web/packages/survival/survival.pdf

17. Newson RB. Comparing the predictive powers of survival models using Harrell's C or Somers' D. *Stata J*. 2010;10(3):339-358.

18. Mallett S, Royston P, Waters R, et al. Reporting performance of prognostic models in cancer: a review. *BMC Med*. 2010;8:21.

19. Altman DG, Royston P. What do we mean by validating a prognostic model? *Stat Med*. 2000;19:453-473.

20. Royston P, Altman DG. External validation of a Cox prognostic model: principles and methods. *BMC Med Res Methodol*. 2013;13:33.

21. Steyerberg EW, Homs MY, Stokvis A, et al. Stent placement or brachytherapy for palliation of dysphagia from esophageal cancer: a prognostic model to guide treatment selection. *Gastrointest Endosc*. 2005;62:333-340.

22. Jatoi I, Anderson WF, Jeong JH, Redmond CK. Breast cancer adjuvant therapy: time to consider its time-dependent effects. *J Clin Oncol*. 2011;29(17):2301-2304.

23. Bland JM, Altman DG. The logrank test. *BMJ*. 2004;328(7447):1073.

CHAPTER 8

Classification Trees and Clustering Algorithms
Danny A. Milner Jr.

▓ INTRODUCTION

Nearly every person can recognize an ancestral chart of either human lineage (as in genealogy) or organism lineage (as in evolutionary biology). Whether the diagram was drawn from physical observations, notes in family documents, or genetic sequencing information, the relationships of individuals in a given diagram are based on a form of collected evidence. In the practice of medicine, a collected group of patients with specific actionable endpoints may need to be differentiated from each other to assign, for example, correct treatment. This is a forward analysis to take the collected data and parse it at points that can be clearly defined. In the science of medicine, cladograms (nonquantitative) and phylogenetic trees (quantitative) are used to show relationships between organisms, strains of bacteria, human-animal homologs, and so on. This is often a reverse analysis where collected data is analyzed backward toward a common ancestor or, more often, an unrelated outlier. For both types of approaches, statistical methods are required to properly place individuals in a given result matrix but also to ensure that the resulting relationships are stable (i.e., statistically significant). In this chapter, approaches to data will be explored with regard to pathology which include classification and regression trees (CARTs) and hierarchical clustering. Other methods for approaching these types of data will also be referred to, albeit in less detail.

■ TOO MANY STAINS!

In the practice of immunohistochemistry, pathologists use a forward-thinking, past-experience-based approach to integrate the histomorphology and clinical history into a panel of stains to confirm their diagnosis. Although the practice has been greatly aided by online databases that can produce panels based on assumptions or produce potential results based on stains, the vast majority of pathologists (and cases) are reduced to a few stains to get to an answer. However, in the areas of hematopathology, soft tissue tumors, or poorly differentiated tumors of unknown primary, the number of stains needed to reach a diagnosis may increase dramatically. After such a difficult case, one might ask, "Is there a better way to do this? Can I get an algorithm?"

Assume a data set exists for 1,000 morphologically similar lymphomas from lymph nodes across the adult age range, which represent 10 unique entities, all of which have a unique single IHC stain that can confirm them. In that setting, for every case, one would have to perform all 10 stains to see which marker was positive for a given tumor (and the diagnostics would be simple but expensive!). But lymphomas share characteristics such as B-cell or T-cell lineage, activation, and so on, and, thus, share staining patterns. When a tumor is CD20 positive (or CD19 positive), one very rarely expects that it would have CD2, CD3, CD5, or CD7 (except aberrantly) because a B-cell lineage is expected. Similarly, one does not expect a CD3-positive cell to express CD20 or CD138. The pathologist's brain is trained to know these associations, but, in aggregate, the logic of how to use the stains in practice may be challenging (especially for trainees!). Going back to the 1,000 lymphomas mentioned earlier, assume now 20 stains (most extraneously) were performed on each case (regardless of the pathologist's input). If the final diagnoses are known (or, e.g., the treatment groups, mortality class), each case can be classified as such (e.g., Burkitt's lymphoma, CHOP, >80% mortality). Assume when the classifications are complete, there are only eight unique groups within the 1,000 samples. One can now ask, retrospectively, "How many stains and in what order do I need to place all 1,000 samples into these eight groups?" The same form of the question could apply to sarcoma (for which a final diagnosis, cytogenetic result, outcome, or gene expression result can be used to classify) or poorly differentiated carcinoma (for which a final organ site, lineage, outcome, or genetic sequence result can be used to classify). The answer lies in the statistical field of decision analysis of which CARTs are one method. There are many others! We focus on CART because it is quite popular in medicine and has free standing software available to perform such analyses with minimal statistical knowledge required.

The basic principle of CART (and similar methods) is sorting. If one starts with 1,000 samples with various shared characteristics of any type (i.e., variables for which each sample has a value assigned and could be categorical or continuous), the samples can be sorted into piles, sub-piles, and sub-sub piles until either there are 1,000 piles (containing one sample each) or there are a reduced number of piles with a set of samples for each (which share some specific characteristic that assigns them to that group). In the previous example, and as is usually the case in these types of analysis, a set number of piles (or outcomes or treatments, etc.) is predetermined and sorting continues until all samples are in one of the piles. If this were an exercise with *actual* patient files, one could imagine sorting by gender, presence of diabetes, presence of hypertension, and history of cigarette smoking into the resulting 16 possible piles (four categorical variables, two possible assignments, $2^4 = 16$). In that exercise, one knows the sorting rules up front and they are discrete. In CART analysis, one does not assume the rules of sorting are known, and they must be empirically determined. If, in the lymphoma example, all 20 stains could be read as simply positive or negative in tumor cells, the number of possible outcomes is 2^{20}, which is greater than 1,000,000 possible results. As only 1,000 lymphomas are included, the possibility of a completely unique result for each case is real but does it have any practical value? Most likely not. Thus, choosing a set of categories at the end (eight groups as earlier) creates a basis for sorting that leads to a practical result. Interestingly, to get to eight groups, one needs three stains at a minimum ($2^3 = 8$), assuming unique discrete staining and an even distribution of a given marker across all lymphomas (which, of course, is not true). Prior to doing any testing, one might hypothesize (or even know from practical experience) that six to eight stains total are needed for classification (with the other 12 to 14 in the data set being either duplication of a similar marker or pathway, constitutive in all lymphomas, or a rare variant that does not impact ultimate outcome).

Figure 8.1 shows an example of how eight classifications (representing 10 entities) can be achieved with only six stains. Note that terminal deoxynucleotidyl transferase (TdT) appears twice in the diagram (depending on B- or T-cell lineage). The endpoints in gray are directly actionable while the endpoints in white require additional information for confirmation, which may be an additional stain or a review of morphologic criteria. CART and other classification methods rely on "gold standard" diagnoses (or categorization) of each sample being used. The

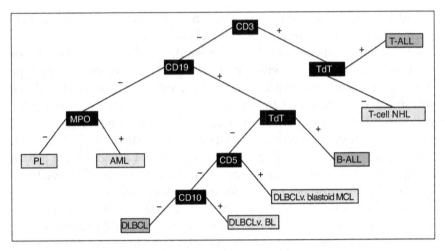

FIGURE 8.1
A tree diagram of immunohistochemical stains for a particular morphological appearance of lymphomas using +/– results in sequence to obtain a diagnosis.

gold standard must be absolute and determined for each case before the analysis is performed. In the case of CART, the algorithm then seeks to minimize the number of nodes (break points) in the tree through comparison of values for a given variable (thresholds). Misclassification of samples can occur in any of these algorithms, and the least number of misclassified with fewest nodes represents the best model.

Some other methods (but not all!) for variable selection in predictive models include support vector machines (SVMs) and elastic nets (ENs). SVMs also employ classification and regression of previously assigned samples but do so as points in space and, thus, can use both linear and nonlinear solutions to produce classification rules. The challenge with SVMs (because of infinite dimensionality available) is overfitting of the primary training data with increased misclassification in the testing data. This is especially true if there are a small number of samples and a large number of variables (as in expression data discussed in the following). EN, on the other hand, is a method which becomes useful in this setting of a large number of predictors in a small sample set (as can be common in gene, transcript, and protein data) (1). EN relies on the correlation between a given variable (e.g., the colinearity) to capture groups of variables together and select predictors and account for all within a given "net" of relatedness (1). Both SVM and EN require advanced statistical knowledge for both preprocessing of a data set prior to analysis as well as executing the analysis because of the number of parameters (inherent to the analytical process) that can be adjusted throughout. Working with a statistician if a model beyond what is possible with CART is required is recommended.

Let's look at a detailed example of CART. Using a hospital records database, a set of patients from emergency room visits are collected from those presenting with "myocardial infarction" (MI) (n = 300), 150 of whom were classified as MI and 150 were found to have other causes for chest pain (noncardiac) (data set online). Minimal data were collected including age (continuous), gender (male = 1, female = 0), other morbidities (diabetes, hypertension, coronary artery disease, all yes = 1, no = 0), smoking history (smoker = 1, nonsmoker = 0), and a C-reactive protein (CRP) value (continuous) from peripheral blood prior to the admission. The researcher wants to know if the data will predict who will have an MI (MI = 1, no MI = 0) based on the data. A CART analysis is performed using CART® within the Salford Predictive Modeler (Salford Systems, San Diego, CA), and the results are shown in Figure 8.2.

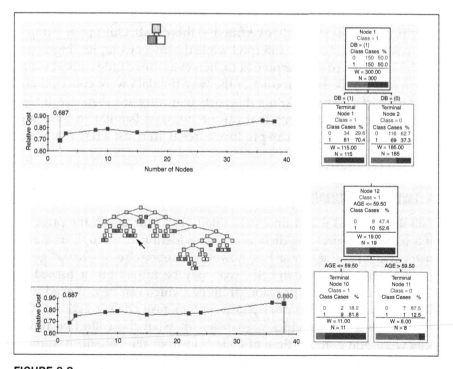

FIGURE 8.2

A set of results from a tree diagram produced by CART software which show the best tree and a classification result (top) as well as the worse tree and an example of a final node (bottom).

Note that within the software, MI will be designated as the target (outcome), and all the other variables are designated as predictors except for patient number, which is excluded. The two outputs shown (left upper and lower) are the trees obtained for the optimal tree (top) and the largest tree (bottom). The optimal tree, in this case, contains a single node which is based on the presence or absence of diabetes. Patients with diabetes (DB = 1) have 70% with MIs while patients without diabetes (DB = 0) have only 37% with MIs (upper right). That does not sound like a very good model, of course, but this is the predicted lowest-cost model of the trees available. The highest-cost model (and largest tree, bottom), has improved prediction (bottom right) and can, for this particular subnode, distinguish 81% with MIs versus 13% with MIs. The criteria (note the arrow in the left lower output), however, are based on age ≤ 59, $7.18 > CRP > 3.89$, in a nonsmoking diabetic patient (whew!). It is clear to see that our gains in classification (or decrease in misclassification) have come at a high cost (in both the model and in the work we have to do to interpret). In addition, it is unlikely that if we tried to implement this model with a new data set that we would get very good classification (this is clearly overfitted to this data!). Our upper (simple, low-cost) model is easy to interpret while the lower (complex, high-cost) model is very hard to interpret; both, however, are of little clinical value, which is most likely a product of the way the data were collected and the design of the study. Within this particular software, there are dozens of parameters and options that can be tweaked (similar to SVM and EN), but the novice user can produce a tree within just a few minutes.

■ TWENTY THOUSAND GENES

Pathologists deal with tumors on a daily basis for which the presence of a handful of proteins dictates a tumor identified through immunohistochemistry. The tumor has, however, a repertoire of ~20,000 genes (just like all other human cells) that may be turned off or turned on at a range of levels. Expression profiling, which can be achieved with RNA sequencing (all transcripts) to polymerase chain reaction (PCR, single transcript), provides a snapshot of what the collective tumor cells were doing at the time of collection from the patient. Assuming that the program of expression harbors unique patterns or combinations of genes, analyzing this data may produce new tumor markers or new pathways for treatment and other interventions. For this type of data (large number of continuous variables), hierarchical clustering is another statistical tool, which arranges the individual tumors by the overall relatedness of the individual gene expression to the total gene expression. The macroscopic heat map that is produced (and plentiful in the literature) gives a snapshot of these groups and the differences between them. How is this heat map generated?

All gene expression data sets generated for publications should be deposited and available on the Gene Expression Omnibus (GEO, www .ncbi.nlm.nih.gov/geo). When you go to the site, the search bar at the top allows you to query any kind of disease you are interesting in reviewing. For example, "Squamous Cell Carcinoma" produces 12,037 resulting entries! One of these, GDS4664, is for lymph-node-positive, early-stage cervical cancer and contains 39 patient samples with expression data performed on the Affymetrix Human Genome U133 Plus 2.0 Array (2). In this study, the TGF-β and β-catenin pathways were shown to be active in metastatic tumors (2). Also in the database, GDS3627 is labeled "Non-small lung cancer subtypes: adenocarcinoma and squamous cell carcinoma" and contains 58 samples (18 SCC and 40 AdenoCA) (3). The original publication of the data shows cell junction differences between the two subtypes based on differential gene expression analysis (3). These are typical examples of manuscript/data sets using expression data. The analysis of expression data can be performed either within a specialized package of software provided by the manufacturer of the expression tool (e.g., Nanostring offers interpretation software for its expression systems), using commercial statistical software with expression packages, or using free online resources that allow for analysis of data (e.g., GenePattern [Broad Institute] or R/Bioconductor) (4,5). The use of GenePattern will be illustrated as a starting point for understanding these analyses, but there are excellent resources on the Internet to learn both systems efficiently and expertly. To begin with GenePattern (after you have picked your favorite data set from GEO), go to: www.broadinstitute.org/cancer/software/genepattern.

The tutorials provided are excellent and cover most of the analyses that a pathologist or laboratory scientist would be interested in seeing. If you have a goal of learning these tools yourself, this is an excellent set of teaching guides for all types of analyses. GenePattern can be used online or you can download the software for offline analysis. You will need to register to use the software but it is freely available after registration. After running through several of the tutorials of interest, browsing through the modules available will give you a sense of the power of the software. The most challenging aspect of using the software is

getting the data into the system correctly. The module called "Prepro-
cess and Utilities" has a tool for getting almost any type of expression
data set into the GenePattern programs. The most useful one is probably the "GEOImporter" which allows any GEO file to be imported and
analyzed by a user. You can select your data set in GEO, download the
".soft" file, convert it with GEOImporter (in GenePattern), and then
follow the manuscript to repeat any analyses that were done. For the
serious student of expression data, this is a fast and efficient way to
familiarize you with this process and have a "hands-on" experience in
doing so.

Back to the concept of a heat map, clustering of this type comes in
several forms, which include supervised clustering and unsupervised
clustering. Which approach is used depends on the type of analysis
planned and includes machine learning, predictive models, and biomarker identification, to name a few. Supervised clustering includes at
the beginning of the experiment all samples (i.e., tumors) being assigned
a classification to a finite number of categories (i.e., in lung, squamous
cell, adenocarcinoma, small cell carcinoma, etc.) in a training set, which
is the equivalent of stating that the categories assigned are the "gold
standard" (6). The clustering algorithm will then organize the genes by
relatedness. A second, new set of samples can then be tested with these
markers and a goodness of fit or classification resulted. This method is
useful for finding biomarkers that describe a special preassigned feature
such as histomorphological classification. This is similar to CART analysis in the assignment of genes to clusters, although the mathematics is
quite different. The obvious problem with this method is, of course, the
initial classification could be incorrect (we assumed we got the "gold
standard" correct).

In the data sets described previously, the data for lung cancers are
an example of supervised clustering where the pathologist has labeled
the case as either adenocarcinoma or squamous cell carcinoma and then
asked what the gene differences were. Because of the variability in differentiation, clinical history, location, and existence of lesions with ques-
tionable morphology, preordained classifications such as this can overly
restrict the data set (requiring "clean" classifications) and reduce the
generalizability of the results.

If, as a pathologist, one considers that the anatomic diagnosis
is based on a collective morphological impression followed by a few
confirmatory proteins (i.e., limited diversity of possible outcomes),

it becomes immediately clear that the diversity attained by ~20,000 variables could produce many additional possible outcomes for the "identity" of a tumor, some of which may share a morphology and a handful of proteins. Thus, a second approach is unsupervised clustering, which does not assume the classification of the samples a priori. In the previous example, depending on how strict the pathologist's histological criteria were, we may get the exact same clusters in supervised versus unsupervised clustering; however, chances are that the unsupervised method would have produce clusters with biologically more related lesions and possibly subsets within a given category because we make no assumptions about the relatedness of the samples. Instead, we look for "natural" or biological classification of the samples based on the relatedness of the overall gene program. The methods by which such clustering is accomplished are variable and include hierarchical clustering (a nearest neighbor tree creation process), partition/centroid algorithms (such as k-means clustering), and many others (6). In this analysis, the data can cluster into physiological expression programs that are similar to each other and produce statistical measures to select the best fit for the number of final categories. One feature of the statistics reported is the cophenetic correlation coefficient (CCC, ranges 0–1), which is a measure of how well a resulted cluster maintains the pairwise distance of the raw data (7). Prior to clustering, one can request that the software produce clustering results or heat maps for any number of clusters and then report a CCC for each—the highest number indicates the best fit.

In Daily et al., a population of patients from Senegal with mild malaria had peripheral blood drawn and the parasites in their blood were analyzed for expression profiles using a *Plasmodium falciparum*–specific Affymetrix array (8). In this data set, no assumptions could be made about the expression profiles of the parasites in a given patient because (a) there was no existing data to compare with other than laboratory experiments, (b) the patients were a heterogeneous mixture of uncomplicated malaria, and (c) the authors wanted to learn something about the biology of the parasites (as opposed to how to classify them). The unsupervised clustering methods in this data set produced three distinct physiological clusters (highest CCC), which, using projection onto existing yeast expression data sets, allowed for classification of these biologies (8). Subsequently, a second set of patients from Malawi with severe malaria were collected and analyzed in the same way (9). The CCC for the final model (0.9853) was for a two-group cluster (k = 2), which demonstrated a strong correlation with parasitemia and a unique physiology not seen in Daily et al. (9). However, the CCC for k = 3, 4, or 5 ranged from 0.9620 to 0.9408, and, most interestingly, when the Malawi data were projected onto the Senegal data, the three Senegal clusters all fell within the smaller Malawi cluster (low parasitemia group) (Figure 8.3, adapted from Daily et al. and Milner et al.) (9).

Thus, having a larger data set in the Malawi group may have easily produced four total clusters if sufficient power had been in the study. In pathology, many similar situations can be imagined where such tools are much more powerful than supervised clustering such as a collection of tumors of unknown primary site, products of conception in spontaneous abortions, bronchoalveolar lavage fluid from patients with a lung mass, or peripheral blood from women under 30 with abdominal pain. In each of these cases, the unsupervised clustering will create natural groups of patients that we can then compare with other clinical data (or, more likely an outcome) or select markers that classify the newly detected groups for better decision making (i.e., procedures to perform, drugs to use, etc.). But, as with any study, the sample size is crucial in making large studies of expression still relatively expensive.

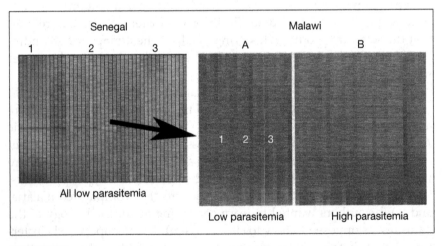

FIGURE 8.3
Two heat maps [review the originals online (9) for better visualization] from two different studies of malaria parasite expression from peripheral blood in a low parasitemia (left) and a low and high parasitemia (right) setting, which demonstrate that the three distinct clusters from Senegal are all found within one cluster from Malawi (the low parasitemia group).

■ CLUSTER COMPLETE . . . NOW WHAT?

Differential Expression Analysis

A question that seems obvious to most observers (and is the lowest-hanging fruit from such an analysis) is simply, "Which genes are over/underexpressed in tumor A versus tumor B?" The implications of such a result could be a new immunohistochemistry marker or biomarker for peripheral blood. Comparing the genes from one tumor to another directly is called differential expression analysis. Mathematically, one is simply asking to find genes that are expressed in both tumors but farthest from each other. This may be absolute (e.g., tumor A has expression of 5,000 units and tumor B has expression of 200 units for a given gene) but assumes that equal amounts of RNA were used in the experiment and that equal proportions of tumor RNA were in the samples. It is thus very easy to understand how, if tumor A was 100% tumor and had 100 micrograms of RNA analyzed versus tumor B was 5% tumor and had 10 micrograms of RNA analyzed, this type of analysis may not be accurate. Another approach is to rank genes from highest to lowest for a given tumor (relative expression) and compare the ranks of the same genes in another tumor (rank order comparison). This type of analysis is less (but still!) affected by absolute expression values or technical problems such as differences in loading, tumor percentage, and RNA degradation. Logically, however, if a gene is ranked first (the most expressed in tumor A) versus 15,000th (in tumor B), the assumption is that the gene is different between the two.

Gene Set Enrichment Analysis

A less obvious question but often more informative than individual gene differences is to determine which groups of genes (or biological pathways) are under- or overexpressed in a given tumor. This can be accomplished through gene set enrichment analysis (GSEA) (10). The goal of GSEA is to look at a collected set of genes associated with a given biological pathway (e.g., DNA synthesis, mitochondrial metabolism, non-Golgi protein export) and ask if the members of that set of genes are present more toward the top or more toward the bottom of an ordered list of genes through a calculated enrichment score (10). Although any one gene may be erroneously overexpressed in a given sample due to a variety of conditions (e.g., mutation, promoters, amplification efficiency, hybridization efficiency, loading RNA quantity), the probability that an entire set of genes in a pathway are all turned on or off is less likely by chance or error. Thus, GSEA allows the investigator to ask what "processes" are at work in this sample and subsequently identify reliable markers for a consistent process that can be practically used.

In Purrington et al., triple negative breast cancers from 704 cases from 10 different studies were analyzed by both unsupervised and supervised clustering as well as gene set enrichment analysis, and then these results were compared with histomorphology and other variables (11). This data set is quite large and the manuscript is massive; however, it pulls together many of the common analyses described earlier (including repetition of previous expression algorithms) and provides a good guide for the pathologist interested in understanding these analyses more fully.

Because, as with any genetic analysis, the system is dealing with large numbers of variables, the threshold for significance is not as simple as a P value of .05. Rather, in GSEA, after normalizing the enrichment scores for the size of a data set, false discovery rate (FDR, less conservative for hypothesis generation) or familywise error rate (FWER, more conservative) can be calculated to determine the "significance" of a gene set in a given sample (10). From a rank ordered list of genes, an enrichment score will reach a point of maximum away from zero (an inflection point), and genes above this threshold are considered to be in the "leading edge" and represent the genes from a given set that are producing the significant enrichment scores (10). The most important consideration in using GSEA on a given data set is the input gene sets and the quality of their annotation. Currently, there are more than 22,000 annotated gene sets available (software.broadinstitute .org/gsea/msigdb/index.jsp), which include hallmark, gene ontology (GO), immunologic, oncogenic, and other gene sets for use in analyzing human and other data (10).

Pathology is a field generating data with enormous amounts of variables for every patient from sodium and hemoglobin to expression levels in tumors. Integration of this data into working models for both providing precision medicine as well as enabling research studies to produce generalized results requires understanding the structure of this data. Even within complex data sets like expression, the structure is still maintained (categorical, continuous, etc.) but the methods of large numbers are required. Categorization approaches and clustering tools allow the pathologist to visualize data structure in an organized way, generate hypotheses about the data and future studies, and, most importantly, provide the best evidence-based decision for a patient's care.

TAKE-HOME POINTS

- Classification (supervised) requires a defined final category for each subject along with a set of variables collected for each subject for predictive modeling.

- Exploratory analysis (unsupervised) of a data set (especially many variables per subject) can produce newly defined categories for each subject.

- Robust methods for small sample sizes with large covariates per sample (e.g., expression analysis) are applications of standard statistics corrected for multiple testing.

QUESTIONS FOR SELF-STUDY

1. How many data sets are there in the GEO for the following diseases: Adenocarcinoma of the cervix? Solitary fibrous tumor? Chromophobe carcinoma? Cardiomyopathy? For accession number GDS4470, how many samples are in the system? How many clusters are evident to you in the heat map? What does the expression of hemoglobin look like in the complete data set (https://www.ncbi.nlm.nih.gov/gds)?

2. A portion of a heat map is shown in the following figure (see following page). Which of the following most likely is true of the data set used to generate this heat map?

   A. The data are a collection of three or more different histological types of lung cancer.

   B. The data are a collection of peripheral blood from a cohort of unselected patients either with or without warfarin treatment.

   C. The data come from a 2:1 male-to-female cohort with the heat map showing activity for a portion of the X chromosome.

   D. The data come from a 4:1 smoker-to-nonsmoker cohort with the heat map showing activity for endothelium-specific genes from the lung at autopsy.

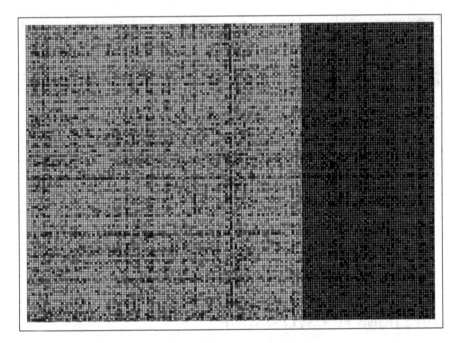

3. Select a manuscript with either classification trees or expression data, obtain the data set from an online resource, and repeat the analysis using a piece of software you have never used before. E-mail me your result!

ANSWERS TO QUESTIONS FOR SELF-STUDY

1. Adenocarcinoma of the cervix = 4. Solitary fibrous tumor = 0. Chromophobe carcinoma = 16. Cardiomyopathy = 41. Note that you can use the "Data set(s)" filter to the top left, which will only give your search results where there are data sets! Samples in glioblastoma study = 46. Number of clusters is ~4. The number of clusters is not clear from this heat map, but there seem to be four distinct regions by eye. For hemoglobin, you need to know the gene name for hemoglobin, which is *HBB* (you can Google it). Then you put that in the "Find gene name or symbol" box at the bottom of the data set's page and hit "Go." The following result is only two clicks away:

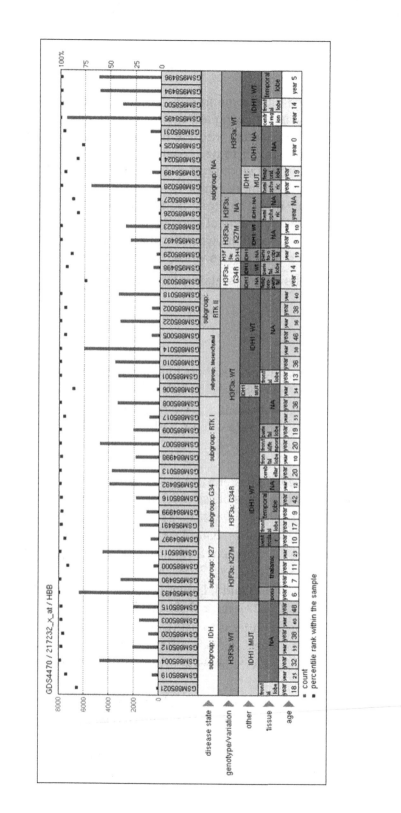

2. Answer: C. The data come from a 2:1 male-to-female cohort with the heat map showing activity for a portion of the X chromosome. Inspecting the heat map shows two distinct clusters, which appear to be present in a 2:1 ratio, so the 4:1 ratio of the smokers would not make sense logically. If the data came from three or more tumor types, we'd expect at least three (probably more) clusters. If the data were from patients on wafarin, we might expect two clusters, but the background physiology of the patients would probably be much more diverse (unselected) so the clusters would not be so tight.

3. E-mail your answers to statsforpath@gmail.com.

■ REFERENCES

1. Zou H, Hastie T. Regularization and variable selection via the elastic net. *J R Statist Soc.* 2005;67(Part 2):301-320.
2. Noordhuis MG, Fehrmann RS, Wisman GB, et al. Involvement of the TGF-beta and beta-catenin pathways in pelvic lymph node metastasis in early-stage cervical cancer. *Clin Cancer Res.* 2011;17:1317-1330.
3. Kuner R, Muley T, Meister M, et al. Global gene expression analysis reveals specific patterns of cell junctions in non-small cell lung cancer subtypes. *Lung Cancer.* 2009;63:32-38.
4. Gentleman RC, Carey VJ, Bates DM, et al. Bioconductor: open software development for computational biology and bioinformatics. *Genome Biol.* 2004;5:R80.
5. Reich M, Liefeld T, Gould J, Lerner J, Tamayo P, Mesirov JP. GenePattern 2.0. *Nat Genet.* 2006;38:500-501.
6. Slonim DK. From patterns to pathways: gene expression data analysis comes of age. *Nat Genet.* 2002;32:502-508.
7. Sneath PH, Sokal RR. Numerical taxonomy. *Nature.* 1962;193: 855-860.
8. Daily JP, Scanfeld D, Pochet N, et al. Distinct physiological states of *Plasmodium falciparum* in malaria-infected patients. *Nature.* 2007;450:1091-1095.
9. Milner DA, Jr., Pochet N, Krupka M, et al. Transcriptional profiling of *Plasmodium falciparum* parasites from patients with severe

malaria identifies distinct low vs. high parasitemic clusters. *PLOS ONE.* 2012;7:e40739.

10. Subramanian A, Tamayo P, Mootha VK, et al. Gene set enrichment analysis: a knowledge-based approach for interpreting genome-wide expression profiles. *Proc Natl Acad Sci USA.* 2005;102:15545-15550.

11. Purrington KS, Visscher DW, Wang C, et al. Genes associated with histopathologic features of triple negative breast tumors predict molecular subtypes. *Breast Cancer Res Treat.* 2016;157(1):117-131.

CHAPTER 9

Dealing With Insufficient and Missing Data
Danny A. Milner Jr.

■ INTRODUCTION

Pathology and laboratory medicine can run the gamut of sample size with some entities in anatomic pathology being seen only a few times a year while some laboratory tests are performed thousands of times per day. For the researcher who chooses to study a rare entity, the challenge of sample size will always be a large one. As finding more samples is not always an option, every effort should be made to utilize these precious samples whenever possible. It is important that a solid understanding of sample size be established as well as a set of tools be available for dealing with missing data.

■ SAMPLE SIZE: HOW MUCH IS ENOUGH?

Much like garlic, one can never have too many samples (or can you?). But the question that constantly plagues a researcher is: "How many is enough samples?" It is crucial to remember that our role in doing an experiment where we are "sampling" a population is that we want whatever we observed to actually have relevance for that population (Figure 9.1).

Take, for example, the following two scenarios.

1. Dr. Johnson observes that calcifications are common in breast lesions and designs a study to see if calcifications on mammogram are associated with breast cancer.

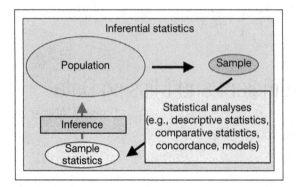

FIGURE 9.1
A model of how inferential statistics are used is shown. A "sample" of the population (our study) is a subset of a larger "population." However large our sample is, the statistics we perform will produce results (means, %, etc.) that we then infer back to the population.

2. Dr. Smith notices that calcifications are common in high-grade phyllodes tumor (when necrosis is present) and wants to design a study to see if such calcifications on mammogram are associated with phyllodes tumor.

Ignoring our bias for this known association, consider the differences in designing a study from the perspective of these two individuals if they had no existing data. Breast cancer is very common, but phyllodes tumor represents less than 1% of cancers. Moreover, high-grade phyllodes tumor with necrosis is even more rare and, in that case, calcifications are probably a consequence of necrosis from a pathway different from the calcifications typically seen in ductal carcinoma. In the first scenario, Dr. Johnson could probably easily design the study to have all mammograms reviewed, scored for calcifications, and then compared to the histology (controlling for some obvious variables). The results of this study may be implications for the population (breast cancer is very common) if Dr. Johnson samples a sufficient number of patients and has sufficient diversity in histological classifications. Dr. Smith, on the other hand, even with a very well-designed study (let's assume the doctor collaborates with 20 cancer centers to find enough cases), may find that calcifications are associated with high-grade phyllodes with necrosis. But how would that knowledge be practically applied? Or another way to ask is: how would this be generalizable to the population? This is not an uncommon problem where researchers may be obsessed with nuance and detail about a particular entity but, in the end, the effect they have measured either is impossible to assess in an efficient way or has no bearing on patient outcome. The important point here is that study design is how we create generalizability. Our observations are crucial to create a hypothesis, but our goal is to sample in such a way as to test that hypothesis as possibly true in the general population.

Sample sizes can be calculated using a range of tools such as the "sampsi" command in Stata (and similar functions in other software) or free online calculators (such as powerandsamplesize.com or a host of others from various universities). Regardless of the calculator, there are several pieces of information that go into the calculations that you need to begin. As long as you have some part of the study design, you can calculate the rest. The important terms (in the case of a t test of means, for example) are the means of the two groups (A and B), the standard deviation (which may be equal or unequal), the sampling ratio (members of A:members of B), power (1—type II error rate or beta), and the significance threshold (type I error rate or alpha) (1). Let's take an illustrative example to understand the challenge at hand.

Consider that we have two groups of autopsy patients who shared a diagnosis of diabetes and hypertension, had an age range of 45 to 70, and were all taking either a calcium channel blocker or a beta-blocker to manage hypertension. Based on selection criteria applied to our search of the medical records, we are examining only patients who had a noncardiac cause of death. Our goal is to measure the thickness of the left ventricle at three different points in comparison with a control measure (a calculation based on the weight and the diameter of the aortic valve) to produce a single continuous variable for each patient which has a dynamic range (based on the limits of mathematics of the equation) from 1.3 to 15.6 and can be accurately and reproducibly measured in a given patient to ±0.2 units (coefficient of variation). Our hypothesis is that the calcium channel blockers reduce hypertrophic effects versus beta-blockers. How many patients do we need in each group? The estimated (or assumed) mean value for a patient in the population is 8.5 ([1.3 + 15.6]/2) if we assume a normal distribution since we know nothing empiric about our measure. The standard deviation could be any number between 0 and 7.2 since we do not know anything about the actual distribution in the population. The following table shows some example sample size calculations assuming the conditions provided:

ASSUMING			RESULTS IN		
MEAN 1	MEAN 2	SD	SAMPLE SIZE	POWER (%)	ALPHA
8.5	10.5	7.2	408	80	0.05
8.5	10.5	1.5	18	80	0.05
3.0	12.0	7.2	22	80	0.05
3.0	12.0	1.5	2	80	0.05

Note that for a measurement that has a tight standard deviation (1.5 vs. 7.2), sample size falls dramatically even when the ranges of the two groups overlap. Note also that when the means are far apart and the standard deviation is tight, any number of samples is sufficient to achieve 80% power at an alpha of 0.05. If we were to increase our power requirement to 99%, we would still only need two samples per group (or four in total) to find the difference significant. When designing this study, however, we have made all of these calculations based on estimates since we have not yet measured the data from our set of hearts. How might we go about determining the range? We do not know if any patient will ever be a 1.3 or a 15.6 in reality, so the mean of 8.5 is totally artificial at this point.

Before selection of any patients, we can take 100 consecutive hearts at autopsy (regardless of history) and measure them along with our other parameters. When we do so, we find that the actual mean for the 100 hearts is 5.7 and the standard deviation is 3.3. In addition, we have three different pathologists measure the same 10 hearts blinded five different times and find that the coefficient of variation is 4% (i.e., repeated measures by the same person do not vary more that 0.2 units). Now we have actual data from which we can calculate a sample size for our study. But, we do not know if our effect will be in one direction or the other or the size of the effect. We can, however, create a new table as follows where we know all variables except sample size (that's being calculated):

ASSUMING			RESULTS IN		
MEAN 1	MEAN 2	SD	SAMPLE SIZE	POWER (%)	ALPHA
5.7	1.7	3.3	22	80	0.05
5.7	2.7	3.3	38	80	0.05
5.7	3.7	3.3	86	80	0.05
5.7	4.7	3.3	342	80	0.05
5.7	6.7	3.3	342	80	0.05
5.7	7.7	3.3	86	80	0.05
5.7	8.7	3.3	38	80	0.05
5.7	9.7	3.3	22	80	0.05

Based on this table, if we have 342 total patients, we will be able to detect a difference of 1.0 unit in our measure with 80% power at an alpha of 0.05. We now do our selection and find that we have 124 patients on a calcium channel blocker and 113 patients on a beta-blocker for a total of 237 patients. Are we sunk since we do not have 342 patients? We can determine this by repeating the calculations with our known sample sizes and asking for the power of our study given an alpha of 0.05 (note that we have all variables in this table except power, which is being calculated).

We can now see that as long as our difference between the two groups is more than two units, we will be sufficiently powered (some would argue "overpowered") to find a significant difference. If we do a little more math (reduce the difference further), we can see that for our sample size, a

ASSUMING			RESULTS IN		
MEAN 1	MEAN 2	SD	SAMPLE SIZE	POWER (%)	ALPHA
5.7	1.7	3.3	124:113	100	0.05
5.7	2.7	3.3	124:113	100	0.05
5.7	3.7	3.3	124:113	99.7	0.05
5.7	4.7	3.3	124:113	64.4	0.05
5.7	6.7	3.3	124:113	66.4	0.05
5.7	7.7	3.3	124:113	99.7	0.05
5.7	8.7	3.3	124:113	100	0.05
5.7	9.7	3.3	124:113	100	0.05

difference of 1.2 more or less than the mean will be powered at 80% to find our difference. Having gone through this, we are confident that our study is powered because we know that the difference is measurable using our scale down to 0.2 units (our low coefficient of variation).

Sample size calculations are becoming an extremely common part of grant applications, which requires familiarity with them. More importantly, however, as in the aforementioned example, performing sample size calculations before you begin collecting data and during the design of a study can insure that the results will be publishable regardless of effect size. A list of the typical types of analyses for which sample size calculations can be performed includes (but is not limited to) (2):

- Test of one mean versus reference value (one- or two-sided *t* test)

- Test of two measured means (one- or two-sided *t* test)

- Test of k (more than two) measured means (analysis of variance [ANOVA])

- Test of one proportion or two measured proportions (binomial proportions)

- Test of survival (time-to-event) data (Cox proportional hazards model)

- Test of odds ratios (ORs) (2 × 2 tables)

Unfortunately, sample size calculations are not possible for all types of analyses. For example, there are no sample size calculators for nonparametric tests. However, a good rule of thumb is that if the parametric equivalent of a nonparametric test is used to calculate a sample size, the power should be sufficient for a nonparametric analysis. Take, for example, the data presented in Figure 9.2.

From the literature, we know the value of procalcitonin for a wild-type mouse with sepsis and for a knockout mouse with the same sepsis model (Figure 9.2, top). We now wish to conduct experiments using a small molecule we hypothesize will interrupt this inflammatory response

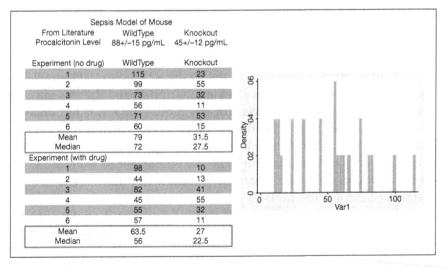

FIGURE 9.2
A mouse model of sepsis using a wild-type mouse and a knockout mouse, both of which are either on or off drug. The raw data are shown on the left for each experiment and a histogram is shown on the right for all of the data combined.

(which we hypothesize will reduce procalcitonin). If we perform a power calculation (for sample size) based on the data from the literature, we would see that we need four animals (two in each group) to detect the same size difference as what we found in the literature (a difference of 43 pg/mL or more). We assume our molecule will have a modest effect, so we only expect a 20 pg/mL difference (or more) is important clinically. Using these numbers would give us a sample size of 16 (that's a lot of mice). For all of these calculations we assume a normal distribution. In our actual data, however, we see that the distribution (given by the histogram in Figure 9.2, right) and the differences in the mean versus the median (Figure 9.2, middle, bottom) suggest these are not normally distributed, so we might choose to use a nonparametric test.

Do we have enough power? In this case, we have two issues. The first is that the actual form of the data is a two-way comparison (mouse and drug) for a single measurement (procalcitonin), which, in normally distributed data, would be a two-way ANOVA. The second is that we are worried that our data is nonnormal and thus we need a nonparametric test. Not only is there not a power calculation possible for nonparametric tests, but there is not a nonparametric equivalent of a two-way ANOVA! So, in this case, we would have to use a two-way ANOVA to test significance specifically with multiple comparison corrections. If we use an estimator for a one-way ANOVA with four comparisons, our sample size needed would be three per group. That's not entirely accurate to our situation but, with six per group, we may be okay.

What happens when we run the analysis? Shown in Figure 9.3 is a plot of the mean and standard deviation (upper) and the median and interquartile range (IQR) (lower) for our mouse data. It is not uncommon to see a figure like this in the literature where a mean and standard error are shown. For the most part, that is inappropriate and probably done to show the "smaller error bars" that occur with a standard error (since it is always smaller than the standard deviation). The goal of a standard error measure is to see how close to the mean in the general population your measure of means falls and accounts for such by numerically dividing by the sample size. In this example, these mice do not exist outside of our experiment so the standard error is really not relevant.

Note that regardless of the display, we can clearly see the effect is due to our existing knockout model and that the drug has had little, if any, effect on either group (the medians for "no drug" vs. "drug" for both mice look to be the same—this is the science of observation). The formal

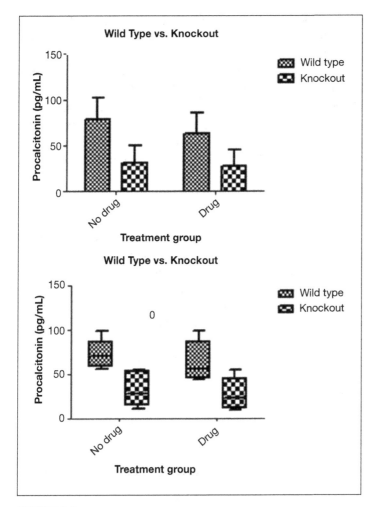

FIGURE 9.3
Two different graphical plots of the mouse data from the experiment
shown as either a mean with standard deviation (top) or a median with
IQR (bottom). Note that with either display, our observation is that the wild
type versus knockout appears to have an obvious effect but the effect of
the drug is not clear.

analysis of the two-way ANOVA demonstrates that 53% of the variation
in the data is explained by "mouse" and only 3% by the "drug." Moreover, the differences between either mouse (drug or no drug) are significant (P value < .05) but there is no difference between drug treatment
(wild type or knockout). But, this is a discussion of power and sample

size. How many samples would we have needed per group to actually see a difference in the mice based on the drug? If we have 24 mice per group with the same distribution of data, the P value for the difference between the wild-type and the knockout mice is now significant (P value .0129) but still accounts for only 3% of the source of variation. Moreover, the effect sizes (16 pg/mL and 4.5 pg/mL) are smaller than we hypothesized would be relevant clinically. Thus, in this example, our initial assumptions for the power calculation were sufficient but our effect size for our hypothesized outcome does not reach a threshold of significance (or clinical relevance).

■ MISSING DATA: WHAT TO DO?

Sample size is a primary consideration when designing a study. During the execution of a study, every effort to collect all data should be used. However, when the data are finally assembled for analysis, it is not uncommon to find a missing value for a given variable for an individual subject. Let's return to the heart measure we discussed previously where we had assembled 237 patients, 124 on calcium channel blockers and 113 on beta-blockers. Remember that all patients had diabetes and hypertension and our age range was 45 to 70. One of the steps in data cleaning is to check for missing data. This can be done by sorting the data by each variable in a spreadsheet or by using a summary feature (Figure 9.4).

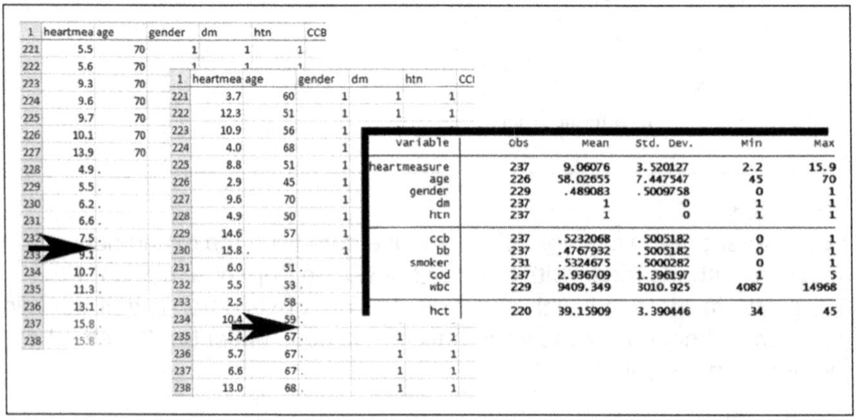

FIGURE 9.4
A screenshot from a spreadsheet showing data sorted by age (far left) with missing values (.), sorted by gender (middle) with missing values (.), and then in a summary table (from Stata) where we can see that not all variables have 237 observations as our main outcome does.

We can see that for our 237 patients, 11 are missing an age value (in the Excel spreadsheet sort on the left). Similarly, we can see that 8 are missing a gender value (in the spreadsheet sort in the middle). A summary for all variables is shown on the right of Figure 9.4 (from Stata). Note that for our variables of interest (heart measure, DM, HTN, CCB, BB, and COD) we have a value for all patients. We have also collected some other variables that might be important, including age, gender, smoking history, white blood cell (WBC) count, and hematocrit (HCT). Note, however, that for all of these variables, we have less than 237 values, which means we have missing data. What can we do?

Drop the Data

If you have the luxury of an enormous database with endless samples, you could choose to simply drop all patients who have incomplete data (although that's probably never a good idea). This is highly dependent on why the data is missing. If we have nonrandomly missing data (e.g., a handful of subjects are missing many values for different variables because of a problem with those subjects), we may simply choose to drop those few subjects if the loss of data is not thought related to the outcome (3–6). If, however, we think the nonrandom loss is explainable by our design (e.g., in a study of schizophrenia spectrum requiring completion of mini mental status exams on follow-up, patients with severe symptoms may be missing as they are less likely to follow up), then we have to account for this missing data (3–6). If we have randomly missing data (e.g., we have missing values for any given variable for any chosen subject without any relationship to other variables for that subject), this may not affect our outcome, but we have to be careful about simply dropping anyone with missing data, as we may reduce our observations and damage our power.

In our heart measure example, if we drop all patients who are missing any data, we are reduced to a total of 187 patients (from 237) (**See online materials; available at www.demosmedical.com/pathology-datasets**). In Figure 9.5, we see that our logistic regression in the table shows the output of a model including all our variables, dropping all patients with missing data (note $n = 187$).

We have OR estimates for each variable in the model and can see we have a value of 0.48 for heart measure with calcium channel blocker (interpreted as each unit decrease in our heart measure values is a 52% reduction in the odds of being on a calcium channel blocker). In Figure 9.5 we see two ROC curves postregression, which show an

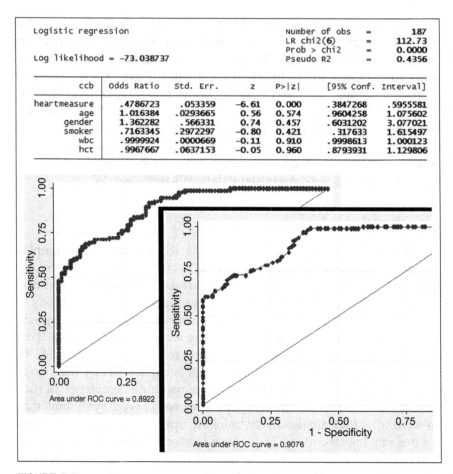

FIGURE 9.5
The results of a logistic regression are shown (top) and then represented as a receiver operating characteristic (ROC) curve graphically (bottom). The left ROC is the complete model and the right ROC is the result of univariate logistic regression with only our heart measure (dropping other variables).

area under the curve (AUC) of 0.8922 for the dropped full model versus an AUC of 0.9076 for univariate regression with all patients (model includes only heart measure). So perhaps dropping these patients was an acceptable method. But we worked hard to measure all those hearts, so how could we reclaim our 50 patients?

Impute Missing Data

Imputation is a powerful tool in many statistical approaches that allows us to put in values for missing variables based on the data that we have. There are many different ways to impute data, but the overall goal is to assign a value to any missing variable so that the subject is not lost from further analysis.

- Impute with replacement—the missing values are replaced with a simple value which could be the mean for all other subjects, a value derived from a regression, an assumption based on the outcome variable, or the last observation duplicated for the next subject (3,4).

- Impute accounting for uncertainty—the missing values are imputed from either multiple imputation or simple imputation with standard error adjustments (3,4,6–8).

- Model the missing values with available data (using assumptions) (3,4,6–8).

In the example of our heart measure, let's look at the variables in detail to see what we could do with a simple imputation method. For age, the mean is 58.03 and the median is 59 (approximately normally distributed). Since we restricted our analysis to patients age 45 to 70, we could use 58.03 as the age for any missing data. If we do that and recalculate, we get a mean age of 58.03 and a median of 58.03 (as we have artificially placed 11 missing values of 58.03 into the data set). This first replacement is simple imputation. If our new mean age had been different from our replacement value, we could replace the ages of those previous missing values with the second mean, and recalculate. We could take the new mean we achieve, substitute, and repeat. This is multiple imputations. For age, at least, this only needs to be done once as the mean has stabilized. Many statisticians recommend at least five rounds of imputation, and others suggest even more (7–9). Note that, for practical purposes, we are reporting age as whole years, so a value of 58 versus 58.03 will likely not affect our outcome or logistical estimates.

What about gender? Gender is a categorical variable (either you are male or you are female in this data set) so imputing a gender isn't as easy as an average. We have 8 missing gender values and our breakdown for the full data set is 117 females and 112 males (51% and 49%).

We could make the assumption that half of the missing data are women and half are men. But how do we assign them to a given existing subject? If we look at our other variables by gender, we can see that, essentially, there is no significant difference between them across the parameters (Figure 9.6).

We can then test the effect of different ways of imputing this variable (a sensitivity analysis) by replacing gender in different ways (Figure 9.6). A t test of means for the missing data versus the assumption about the size of women's hearts (as well as all replacements shown) is greater than 0.05, suggesting whichever we choose will probably not affect our outcome (all forms of imputed data are equivalent with regard to our outcome).

Missing Data:

gender	mean(heartm~e)	mean(age)	mean(wbc)	mean(hct)
0	9.12308	58.1893	9686.74	39.0642
1	9.15089	57.6266	9206.78	39.4563

All male assigned to missing:

gender	mean(heartm~e)
0	9.12308
1	9

All female assigned to missing:

gender	mean(heartm~e)
0	8.98
1	9.15089

Alternating assignment (start with women = 0, then 1, 0, 1, 0, 1, 0, 1 on left below) or alternating assignment (start with men = 1, then 0, 1, 0, 1, 0, 1, 0 on right below)

gender	mean(heartm~e)
0	8.99091
1	9.13362

gender	mean(heartm~e)
0	9.10744
1	9.01207

Assume women's hearts are smaller, on average, than men's (assign four smallest numbers to women and four largest numbers to men)

gender	mean(heartm~e)
0	8.97934
1	9.14569

FIGURE 9.6

An exploratory analysis of what happens to the mean heart measure when we use different methods of assigning missing gender.

We can apply similar corrections to the variables for smoker, WBC, and HCT (the latter two similar to age) and then repeat the logistic regression for our univariate and multivariate models (Figure 9.7).

For the univariate model (as before) we get an AUC of 0.9076 and with the inclusion of all our data (none are missing after imputation) we get an AUC of 0.9126. Note that our univariate logistic, multivariate logistic (missing), and multivariate logistic (imputed) estimated ORs for our heart measure are 0.45, 0.48, and 0.45, all significant in all models. Thus, by having a larger sample and including all subjects, we hope our model is more robust and our OR estimate more accurate.

As a rule of thumb, the first attempt to replace missing data should be to actually go back to the experiments or original data collection process

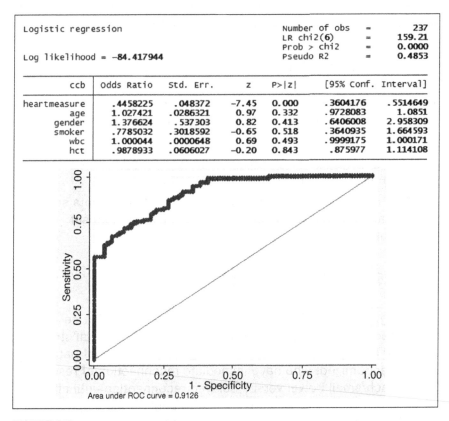

Logistic regression

		Number of obs	=	237
		LR chi2(6)	=	159.21
		Prob > chi2	=	0.0000
Log likelihood = −84.417944		Pseudo R2	=	0.4853

ccb	Odds Ratio	Std. Err.	z	P>|z|	[95% Conf. Interval]	
heartmeasure	.4458225	.048372	−7.45	0.000	.3604176	.5514649
age	1.027421	.0286321	0.97	0.332	.9728083	1.0851
gender	1.376624	.537303	0.82	0.413	.6406008	2.958309
smoker	.7785032	.3018592	−0.65	0.518	.3640935	1.664593
wbc	1.000044	.0000648	0.69	0.493	.9999175	1.000171
hct	.9878933	.0606027	−0.20	0.843	.875977	1.114108

Area under ROC curve = 0.9126

FIGURE 9.7
A repeat logistic regression now with all of the variables included because we have imputed all missing values. Note that the ROC curve has improved and our estimate of heart measure is stable.

and retrieve these numbers. If there is a need to impute data (i.e., it can't be found or regenerated), always state in the methods section exactly what was done and what assumptions were utilized for any imputation performed. Except when the data are simple, as in our examples, it is always best to consult with a statistician if significant imputation is required to salvage a data set. These individuals have a range of tools and approaches (partial imputation, partial deletion, expectation–maximization algorithm, interpolation, and complex model-based techniques). If possible, a sensitivity analysis (similar to the exercise with gender in Figure 9.6 but actually going to the full model) should be performed to make sure the boundaries of the assumptions do not greatly change the results. Any manuscript which uses imputed data should explicitly discuss this in the paper and address any results for sensitivity analysis or other boundaries of the result that should be considered by readers.

TAKE-HOME POINTS

- Sample size and power calculations are crucial components for both planning a study (budget, resources, etc.) and reporting an actionable result (not overpowering).
- Missing data, when possible, should be located at the data source and original data should be used.
- When data are missing and cannot be found at the data source, imputation methods can be used to complete a data set, assuming certain rules are followed.

QUESTIONS FOR SELF-STUDY

1. A surgical colleague approaches you about a study to be conducted involving patients who have gastrointestinal stromal tumor (GIST) aimed at understanding the outcomes of patients (nonrandomized) who have immediate reconnection of resected stomach/small bowel versus delayed reconnection until after chemotherapy. You would be asked to confirm the diagnosis of GIST by immunohistochemistry and exclude other entities that would not receive the same chemotherapy. The outcome the surgeon is most concerned with is breakdown of surgical site. What are your concerns with such a study?

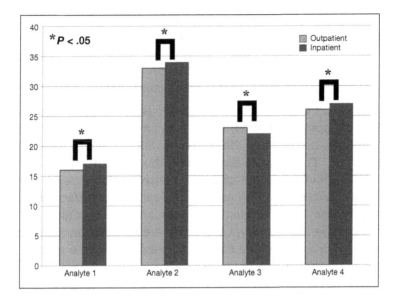

2. A clinical study requires chemistry data from your laboratory analyzer, which is downloaded daily for 6 months to a database to select patients who are admitted to hospital versus outpatients. The analyzer records, for each patient, the single highest value for four different analytes. You get a preliminary data analysis from the research team as shown in the chart. How do you respond to these data?

3. As part of a quality control (QC) project for your hospital, you are working with a team of three people to analyze a data set collected from all patients having a core needle biopsy over a 2-year period with follow-up information. One of the variables is the ICD-10 code for the surgical resection following the core biopsy, and you note that 35% of the patients are missing this value. What do you think about that?

ANSWERS TO QUESTIONS FOR SELF-STUDY

1. In this particular study description, the sample size is likely to be very small overall (incidence of GIST), be unbalanced (patients are not randomized so there is no way to be sure you have equal numbers of the two interventions), and have few comparators

(surgical site complications are also rare). Most importantly, without randomization, most surgeons will elect to do what they think is safe based on the literature, so the numbers of patients in a given group will be skewed by the surgeon performing the procedure, introducing another bias (surgeon).

2. The data set described must have thousands of samples, given the commonality of the analytes measured, and, thus, any difference between the values would appear statistically significant. The main challenge with the data, as reported, is that the effect sizes (the difference between the measures for inpatient and outpatient) are not clinically relevant/actionable although they reach statistical significance. This is an example of overpowering a study. Last, there are no error bars (standard deviation or interquartile range), so we don't have a sense of how variable the data are overall.

3. The variable that is missing is an ICD-10 code for patients who had a surgical resection. In this case, the first procedure was a core needle biopsy, which may have shown a malignant or benign result. Benign results would most likely not have a follow-up surgery and, thus, not have a second ICD-10 code. In addition, patients may have been lost to follow-up (regardless of the primary diagnosis). Last, the ICD-10 code could have just been forgotten in the data collection. Thus, these data are nonrandom missing data (we can easily explain why they are missing) and, thus, we would need to account for this in the analysis (or else lose patients). To begin, we should check all patients missing second ICD-10s to see if there is a data point in the clinical record. For patients lost to follow-up, we could consider using the ICD-10 from the primary core biopsy unless part of our study is based on concordance of biopsy and resection (in that case, we would probably have to exclude them). For the benign diagnoses seen on the core, we can use the same code for the missing data with a note that we had to duplicate the code because of a lack of procedure which was not clinically indicated.

■ REFERENCES

1. Power and Sample Size. Available at powerandsamplesize.com
2. Tu W. Basic principles of statistical inference. *Methods Mol Biol.* 2007;404:53-72.

3. Cochrane Handbook for Systematic Reviews of Interventions. Available at www.cochrane-handbook.org

4. Roderick JA, Rubin DB. *Statistical Analysis with Missing Data.* 2nd ed. Hoboken, NJ: Wiley-Interscience; 2002.

5. Rosner B. *Fundamentals of Biostatitics.* 6th ed. Belmont, CA: Duxbury; 2006.

6. Van den Broeck J, Cunningham SA, Eeckels R, Herbst K. Data cleaning: detecting, diagnosing, and editing data abnormalities. *PLOS Med.* 2005;2:e267.

7. Graham JW, Olchowski AE, Gilreath TD. How many imputations are really needed? Some practical clarifications of multiple imputation theory. *Prev Sci.* 2007;8:206-213.

8. Rubin DB. *Multiple Imputation for Non-Response in Surveys.* New York, NY: Wiley; 1987.

9. Vach W, Blettner M. Biased estimation of the odds ratio in case-control studies due to the use of ad hoc methods of correcting for missing values for confounding variables. *Am J Epidemiol.* 1991;134:895-907.

Index

Printed in the United States
By Bookmasters